The Bullet's Yaw

The Bullet's Yaw

✦

Reflections on violence, healing and an unforgettable stranger

Dustin W. Ballard, MD

iUniverse, Inc.
New York Lincoln Shanghai

The Bullet's Yaw
Reflections on violence, healing and an unforgettable stranger

iUniverse books may be ordered through booksellers or by contacting:

iUniverse
2021 Pine Lake Road, Suite 100
Lincoln, NE 68512
www.iuniverse.com
1-800-Authors (1-800-288-4677)

Because of the dynamic nature of the Internet, any Web addresses or links contained in this book may have changed since publication and may no longer be valid.

The views expressed in this work are solely those of the author and do not necessarily reflect the views of the publisher, and the publisher hereby disclaims any responsibility for them.

ISBN: 978-0-595-47648-0 (pbk)
ISBN: 978-0-595-91911-6 (ebk)

Printed in the United States of America

Contents

Acknowledgments

First and foremost, I'd like to express my immense gratitude to Jeffrey Mains; not only for allowing me to investigate his story but also for encouraging me to tell it. Jeffrey, I appreciate your honesty, patience, persistence and friendship. Thanks also to Linda Mains for providing so many details of her and her son's ordeal. I am certain that re-living it all was not easy for either of you and I thank you both for having the courage to do so. I'd also like to express my appreciation to all of my colleagues at UC Davis Medical Center and specifically those who helped guide and inform this manuscript: Drs Garen Wintemute, David Wisner, William Blaisdell and Mark Borden. Also, many thanks to friends and family who were patient enough to read and provide feedback on the multiple iterations of this book: Chris and Alexandra Ballard, Phil and Roberta Ballard, Beth and Mel Keiser, Erik Larson, Ryan and Jodie Craig, Melissa Murphy, Sam Jackson and Julian Husbands. I am particularly grateful also to John A Ware, whose willingness to repeatedly read my work helped drive it forward. And the greatest thanks go to my wife Angela, for her endless encouragement and assistance.

I'd be remiss if I didn't thank the thousands of patients who I have seen and treated in EDs throughout Northern California; interactions with these patients have provided much of the tissue of this book. In many cases, I have modified names, descriptions and circumstances to protect their privacy. And while they may never know it, every one of them has helped me to become a better physician.

Visit my blog at:
http://incisionanddrainage.blogspot.com/

Snapshots

During my three-year residency in emergency medicine I treated thousands of patients—strangers about whom I learned intimate details. Most passed through my life swiftly and the circumstances of their illnesses left but a wisp in my memory. A handful of patients, however, marked me forever. *The Bullet's Yaw* is the story of one of these unforgettable strangers and what he taught me about life, violence and healing.

When I tell people what I do for a living, I often get responses along the lines of "Wow, good for you … you must have some great stories," or "ER, huh? I bet you see some crazy injuries and stuff." And it's true, I do and I have. There are a dozen or so morbidly fascinating tales that I can recite to appease curiosity. These go-to stories of mine summon the bizarre and grotesque and are like mean political ads—loud, obnoxious and mercifully short. For instance, I might recount the time that a dirty and disheveled man asked me to retrieve a Geiger counter from his rectum, explaining that it was placed there in 1963, by his father, by the order of the U.S. Supreme Court. Or the day that I treated an elderly heroin junkie from a squalid housing project who arrived in the emergency department (ED) barely coherent and completely unaware that his feet were teeming with maggots. Or perhaps I'd describe a Folsom Prison inmate with a penchant for self-mutilation who needed multiple razor blades extracted … from his penis' urethra. Usually, these stories, and others like them, are good for an immediate gape or guffaw followed by wordless acknowledgment that my job is not to be envied. Every once in a while the listener will ask how it all turned out, with a query like "The guy with the maggots, what happened next? Did he ever return to a normal life?" Until recently, my answer to such questions had always been "I don't know."

As an emergency physician, my job is full of snapshots—of lives and illnesses—and I am professionally rewarded less for the richness or resolution of these snapshots than for the quantity. The field of emergency medicine is ripe with terms that describe the transitory nature of our patient interactions, some academic (throughput) and others colloquial (move the meat). For many emergency physicians like me, "throughput" was one of the primary reasons we chose the field. When I go to work, I go for a discrete amount of time and I start from scratch. This makes my experience different from most physicians, who have a panel of patients or an operating room schedule or are shackled to their pagers and never sure when duty will call. I work shifts, the length and time of day varies (some are eight-hour shifts, some twelve-hour shifts, some normal business hours, and some graveyard) but the duration of my duty is pretty much set in advance. Just about everything else about my work, on the other hand, is both unpredictable and fleeting. The vast majority of patients I treat I will never see again. They arrive in the emergency department, are seen and either admitted to the hospital, transferred to another facility, or discharged home. Perhaps this process takes five minutes, perhaps it takes several hours, but all of the patients move on, to be replaced by others. Much of the work becomes rote, and most of these patients are, by necessity, forgettable.

For the most part, I relish the brevity of my clinical encounters. Many patients have a fixable problem, such as a dislocated finger or simple laceration, and can be quickly put back together. Other clients test my nerves with a litany of chronic complaints and I am thankful that I need only address the most pressing ones and then refer the patient elsewhere. There are occasions, however, that I wish there was more continuity to my job and that some of my snapshots could be spliced together into a film. As I've progressed beyond residency and into the full time profession of emergency medicine, such moments have become more common, and my desire to produce a more lasting body of work has grown stronger. And that is why I decided to tell this story. *The Bullet's Yaw* is about a memorable patient—a patient who I treated in residency whose story resonated with me, and who, years later, I sought out to answer the question "What happened next?" Finding the answer enriched me in ways I wouldn't have predicted and I hope that this story will do the same for you.

1

Hank Doe

"I giveth and I taketh … that's how it goes in (expletive) life. I put on a hell of a show. I've taken four victims; this should be good enough to last about a week on the news. It's time to feed the news media … I'm going down in (expletive) history."

—Excerpts from Joseph Ferguson's video tape,
filmed September 9th, 2001

"A man simply in the wrong place at the wrong time. Shot while sitting at a stoplight in his pick-up truck."

—From Sacramento News 10, September 10th, 2001

At first, two minutes per day was all I budgeted for Jeffrey Mains. Two minutes—about the length of an on-the-go shower, a pre-flight safety video or the morning line at Starbucks. Two minutes dedicated to a job is hardly ever enough to feel that the task has been performed thoroughly. But as a moist-behind-the-ears intern on the Trauma Surgery "Gold" team at the UC Davis Medical Center (UCDMC) in Sacramento, in charge of 30 or more convalescing patients, that was all I could afford. Or at least, several months removed from medical school and with a seemingly endless daily checklist of clinical errands, it sure seemed that way. The arithmetic was simple; I had an hour to do my morning patient rounds in the Trauma Nursing Unit (which I knew simply as the TNU) and with 30 patients or so to round on, that worked out to about two minutes each. When I look back, I am not surprised that my daily litany of tasks—recording vital signs, writing progress notes and admission orders, adjusting medications, changing wound dressings, checking chest tube drainages, harassing the radiologist to read x-rays, answering nursing questions and dictating discharge summaries—overwhelmed and stifled my curiosity. I cognitively coded my patients with one-line clinical descriptions such as "32-year-old male status post-fall with right-

1

sided rib fractures," and pertinent clinical data such as "chest x-ray negative for lung injury." For the most part, I knew only snippets of their life stories and was better equipped to recite daily surgical drain output than marital status. The situation with Jeffrey Mains was different. Unlike many of the tenants of the TNU who were trauma patients with uncomplicated injuries or surgical patients who had turned the corner, twenty-seven year-old Jeffrey Mains was well into a prolonged hospitalization filled with setbacks. Trauma victims without serious injury were often in and out of the TNU in 24 hours; it had taken Mains 23 days just to make it out of the Surgical Intensive Care Unit (SICU). And there was also his celebrity status—a survivor of one of the deadliest shooting sprees in California's history—and a front-page name for two days until the events of September 11th swept him to the back pages. I knew the basics of the story, everyone in the hospital had heard about the security guard who went psycho and the innocent bystander whom he nearly killed. So Jeffrey Mains could and should have piqued my interest. But I only had two minutes.

Jeffrey Mains shared a room with Mr. Wellburn, a middle-aged African-American with an inflamed pancreas brought on by excessive boozing. Mr. Wellburn was on "bowel rest" and was being treated with intravenous fluid and pain medication until his pancreas settled down and he could safely eat again. He was also bored with his hospitalization so he liked to pull stunts, like stealing snacks from other patients and smoking cigarettes in the bathroom. On the third day of his hospital stay, Mr. Wellburn disappeared without notice and with his intravenous line (IV) still in place. I spent several hours trying to track him down, finally reaching him by phone at home. He told me that he had left to get some proper clothing and that he would return soon. True to his word, he arrived back at the TNU in a 1970's gold zoot suit, replete with bell bottoms. "If yur gonna make me stay here," he said, "I might as well be pimpin'."

Each morning, between 4 and 5, I'd swing into their room for approximately four minutes. My interactions with Mr. Wellburn were unpredictable—I was never sure what I'd find in his hospital bed. One morning all I saw was dark braided hair resting on the covers and was surprised to discover that it belonged not to my patient, but to a girlfriend visiting for the night. My interactions with Jeffrey Mains, on the other hand, were more rote. I'd ask him a few questions: "Are you having any pain?" "Are you having any difficulty breathing?" "Have you felt nauseous or vomited?" "Did you eat anything yesterday?" "When was the last time you passed gas?" and receive short answers. Then I'd place my stethoscope briefly on his chest, my hands on his abdomen, and sweep out of the room. I never had the time to ask detailed questions or to learn about his life before September 9th, 2001. I didn't know that he'd been working for a year and a half as a plumber's apprentice with the local 447 and that he'd recently decided to pursue a career in plumbing. I didn't know that he'd spent four years in the military and done a tour of duty in South Korea as a heavy-equipment mechanic. I had no idea that he'd been devastated when his dad left to start a new family with a different woman and that he'd struggled with bouts of heavy drinking that only stopped when his mom issued an ultimatum. I could have guessed that he was close to his mother (Linda) and his uncle (Gary), because the TNU nurses told me that they visited every day, but I had no idea how strong those bonds were. I certainly would have been surprised to learn that he had a passion for art and that he spent his free time, when not playing pick-up basketball or hanging with his friends from Christian Brothers High School, visiting the Crocker Art Museum or working on charcoal still lifes. Or that his dream was to one day teach art at the college level. And it wasn't until years later that I learned that he had a serious girlfriend but that it was another woman, who had married someone else while Jeffrey was in the military, who frequently visited him in the hospital. It wasn't that I didn't empathize with Mains. On the contrary, we were both in our late twenties and I sensed that he was a gentle and generous soul; under different circumstances we may have become friends. But, necessity (or perceived necessity) dictated that my knowledge of him be mostly numerical and heavily formulaic.

Several hours after my pre-dawn visit, I'd return to Mains' room with the Trauma Gold team—a crew of doctors and students led by our attending physician, the chief of trauma surgery, Dr. David Wisner. During this second visit I'd regurgitate information: "Jeffrey Mains is a 27-year-old status post gunshot wound to the abdomen with a complicated post-op course, now on Hospital Day number 40. His temperature this morning was 98.5, his BP was 125/84, heart rate 75 and respirations 16. His ins and outs were 4400 over 3100, including 10cc out of his Jackson Pratt drain. His exam is unchanged." Dr. Wisner would nod knowingly and say a few encouraging words to Mains and then a few of firm direction to me before leading our pack briskly to the next room. Several times, I caught Dr. Wisner taking an extra look at Mains, an empathic look. In retrospect, I suppose this was because, even with all he'd seen during a long career as a trauma surgeon, Mains' story was particularly unfortunate and his recovery had been particularly complicated.

Every morning, when I came by for my allotted two minutes and asked Jeffrey Mains what was bothering him, I received familiar answers. He was "restless," "hurting," "frustrated." And there were even darker days, days when I got the sense that Mains wished that he had died, that the emergency response hadn't been so fast or the surgery expedient. He was 27, brutally scarred across his chest and abdomen, confined to his hospital bed and unable to eat anything other than ice chips. Even though his physical survival had been miraculous, he didn't know how to process the randomness of his injury or the uncertainty of his future. For Jeffrey Mains, everything had changed in a moment of senseless violence. Years after first meeting Jeffrey Mains I went searching for the details of that moment, and this is the story I found.

◆   ◆   ◆

Joseph Ferguson had a simple agenda and it was "to go down in fucking history." "I giveth and I taketh away," he proclaimed in a six-minute video filmed behind barricaded doors on September 9th, 2001, "that's how it goes in fucking life."

Twelve hours earlier, in the dim glow of the setting moon, twenty-year-old Joseph Ferguson had begun his quest for immortality. Ferguson spent the pre-dawn hours firing off rounds at a shooting range and then donned military fatigues and a bullet-proof vest and loaded his car with an AK-47 assault rifle, a 9mm handgun, a sawed-off shotgun, and more than 150 rounds of ammunition. Distraught over a recent break-up with his girlfriend and dissatisfied with his job at Burns Security in Sacramento, he then shot and killed four people, including his ex, Nina Susu. He used his cellular phone to warn and taunt his co-workers and soon-to-be victims. To some, he bragged that he planned to "outdo Soltys," referring to Nikolay Soltys, a Ukrainian immigrant who, just weeks prior, had killed his wife and unborn child along with five other family members.[1]

Ferguson's homicidal mission took him to the Miller Park Marina where he gunned down two more people and then to the Land Park Zoo, where he accosted a female Burns employee at gun point. He took her car keys and left her unhurt and handcuffed to a railing near the emu exhibit. Law enforcement officers were frantic. "This is [my] worst nightmare," sheriff's captain John McGinness told the *Sacramento Bee*.

Next, Ferguson traveled to the Rancho Cordova house of his former co-worker, Nikolay Popovich. There, he held Popovich and his wife Lyudmilla hostage, forcing them to feed him, help him barricade their house against the police, and film his video. "I put on a hell of a show," he boasted. "I've taken four vic-

---

1.   Sacramento police had recently found Soltys, barefoot and brandishing a metal potato peeler, under a desk in his mother's home in nearby Citrus Heights.

tims … that should be good enough to feed the news media." Not long after finishing his film, at around 9pm, Ferguson raised the death tally to five—executing Nikolay Popovich with a single bullet to the back of the head. Lyudmilla Popovich was supposed to be next but, for reasons that we will never know (perhaps because she read to him from the Bible), Ferguson didn't kill her. Instead he left his make-shift bunker and drove the couple's dark blue Nissan several miles away to a quiet section of Goethe Road where he left Lydumilla unharmed and in possession of his videotape. Several hours later, after having received Lydumilla's 9-1-1 call, police identified the stolen vehicle traveling near Zinfandel and International Drives.

At an intersection on Zinfandel, two California Highway Patrol vehicles pulled up next to the dark blue Nissan. Without warning, a thin man in fatigues emerged from the vehicle and opened fire with an AK-47 assault weapon. It was a brief and mostly one-sided exchange of gunfire and, after wounding a CHP officer, Joseph Ferguson jumped back in the Nissan and barreled away. At the intersection of Zinfandel and Folsom, he crashed into a fire hydrant, stepped out of the car and resumed firing. Behind him, in a Jack in the Box parking lot, patrons sprinted for safety as Ferguson wildly fired off more than 100 rounds of ammunition, peppering the ground and vehicles with bullets and blowing out patrol car windows. "It was like a war" said an on scene police detective. Then, perhaps sensing a new police presence, Ferguson turned and directed his weapon at a pick-up truck.

Jeffrey Mains was driving his white Toyota 4x4 truck to the corner grocery store to get a can of chew. It was a little before midnight on a quiet Sunday evening, and the heat of the day was finally dissipating. Mains had spent the day relaxing with his sister, who was visiting from Los Angeles, and his mother Linda. After his sister had flown home in the evening, he returned to his Rancho Cordova apartment. He was due at the local 447 early the next morning but wasn't particularly tired and needed a fix of chewing tobacco. As he stopped at a traffic light at the intersection of Zinfandel Drive and Folsom Boulevard, he flipped on his left blinker. On the radio, news reporters may have been discussing the day's downtown shootings and perhaps comparing them to the Nikolay Soltys murders. Or maybe they were talking about Barry Bonds, and the record-setting three home runs he'd hit that night for the San Francisco Giants. Jeffrey Mains can't remember because he wasn't listening; he was distracted by a sudden commotion.

It happened so fast that Jeffrey Mains had no idea what had hit him. A hollow point bullet fired from an AK-47 assault weapon and traveling at 1500 feet per second ripped through the door of his truck and struck him in the left flank. The bullet's path through steel slowed its velocity, which was bad news for Mains because it meant that when the missile collided with him it didn't pass straight through, but instead tumbled sideways, a phenomenon that ballistics experts call the bullet's yaw. Conventional AK-47 bullets are designed to minimize yaw and stay true to their course for 30 to 40 centimeters after entering human tissue, which considering that the average human trunk is 40 centimeters thick, means that AK-47 wounds are typically clean and uncomplicated—but not the wound to Jeffrey Mains. The bullet's impact and subsequent yaw, according to veteran trauma surgeon William Blaisdell, must have been "like an explosion," creating a cavity (30 times the diameter of the bullet) that undulated for several fractions of a second before collapsing. The moment of energy transfer was over in a blink, but the anatomical damage would last much longer. Mains' bowel was pierced and leaking in multiple locations, his liver was lacerated and his right diaphragm ruptured. A section of his small intestine spilled outside his abdominal wall and blood pooled in his peritoneal cavity. His peripheral blood vessels constricted, diverting blood to his vital organs and causing his skin to mottle. Jeffrey Mains was in shock—not only psychologically stunned from the swiftness of his injury, but also physiologically reeling from a rapid loss of blood. Very slowly, he opened his truck's door, stumbled out, attempted to take a few steps and collapsed in the middle of the road.

Off-duty sheriff Craig Hill heard reports of a gun fight on his police radio and drove to the scene—where he saw a young man with a basketball player's build slumped on the asphalt in open view of a man with an assault weapon. Someone yelled, "He's been shot, he's been shot," and during a brief pause in the firefight Hill pulled his Chevy Tahoe in front of the victim, absorbing a bullet in his bumper. "There's no way I could wait and watch [him] die in front of us," he later told reporters. With the Chevy shielding him, Hill and two other officers, including sheriff's deputy Rhea Pelster, pulled Jeffrey Mains into a patrol car and radioed for an ambulance. "When I first got there," Pelster told the *Sacramento Bee*, "[Mains] wanted his hand held. I could tell he was slipping rapidly away from us. The more I held his hand, the wetter and colder it was becoming. He was going to die if he stayed there much longer."

Minutes later, the thumping of gunfire stopped. Officers cautiously moved in on the Nissan. In the front seat they found Ferguson, shot in the chin at close range with a 9mm. He'd kept the promise he'd made to his video camera to "just pop" himself.

The paramedics of Sacramento Fire ambulance M31 arrived on scene at 12:08am to find a mottled and sweat-coated Jeffrey Mains. Their "patient care report," often called the "run report," noted an approximately 2-inch section of eviscerated bowel (bowel protruding beyond the skin) without external bleeding. The victim's systolic blood pressure was recorded as 80 (normal is 110-140) and his heart rate was 120 (normal is 60-100). Unit M31 loaded him into their ambulance and turned on the lights and sirens, traveling "Code 3," the highest priority of emergency medical transport, to Sacramento County's premier trauma center. En route to UC Davis Medical Center (UCDMC), the medics worked rapidly as Mains' consciousness waxed and waned. He was placed on an electronic heart monitor and intravenous catheters were inserted in each forearm with the saline running "wide open." Mains received oxygen through a face mask at a rate of 15 liters a minute. Eleven minutes later, with red lights blaring and sirens calling, Unit M31 pulled into the ambulance bay.

In the trauma bay of the UC Davis emergency department (ED),[2] a specialized team, many of them dressed in baby-blue plastic gowns and wearing clear face shields, huddled around an empty gurney. The hospital operator had paged the most urgent of trauma codes, a "911," and all over the hospital, specialists dropped what they were doing and hurried to the ED. Just outside the trauma bay, on the triage whiteboard in the long corridor that connects the ambulance bay to the ED and the main hospital, a scribbled note read "27 yo male. GSW to abd. BP 80/P. 2 IV's. ETA 8 min." At the registration desk an identification card, bracelet and lab stickers were being printed. Later, the patient's real name would be registered, but for now he was *Hank Doe*.

The chief of trauma surgery, Dr. David Wisner, stood in the trauma bay, as did the trauma fellow, the senior surgical resident, a junior surgical resident, and two interns.[3] The emergency physician on-duty was also there with his senior resident. An x-ray technician was on hand and an ultrasonographer en route. A handful of nurses were positioned throughout the room: one to "scribe" notes, one to check blood pressure, and two to assess IV placement and hang fluids. The operating room was on alert.

---

2.   Thanks in part to the popularity of the television show "ER," most Americans are more familiar with this term than "ED." Within the emergency medicine community, however, the preference is for emergency department (ED)—a term that incorporates the specialized nature of the care facilities and recognizes that virtually every "ER" contains more than one room.

3.   The medical training hierarchy goes as follows: Lowest is the *intern* who is fresh out of medical school, next is the *junior resident*, then the *senior resident*, and finally the *fellow* who is one-notch below an *attending* physician.

Once the paramedics wheeled Jeffrey Mains through the pneumatic sliding doors of the ED, a well-practiced protocol, that to the untrained eye might seem like coordinated mayhem, was initiated. As the medics gave a verbal report, they transferred Mains onto a gurney. Nurses and doctors swooped in, cutting off his clothes with trauma shears and applying a blood pressure cuff to his right arm, stickers and leads for a cardiac monitor to his chest, and an oxygen saturation monitor to his index finger. With the captain of the ship, Dr. Wisner, observing silently from the back of the room, the senior emergency medicine resident assessed the airway. The resident asked the patient what his name was and must have received an acceptable answer, because the ED record notes that "Hank Doe" was breathing on his own and answering questions appropriately. Several doctors listened to his chest to ensure that both lungs were inflating and exhaling equally. Within fifteen seconds the A (Airway) and B (Breathing) of the well-established ATLS (Advanced Trauma Life Support) A-B-C-D-E algorithm had been assessed and E (Exposure) was already in progress. The C (Circulation) was evaluated by checking Mains' blood pressure and pulse and the D (Disability) assessed by having him wiggle his toes. His blood pressure was 70/p, about half of normal, but he maintained adequate peripheral pulses. His engine was strong but his tank was nearly empty—the bleeding had to be stopped. Jeffrey Mains spent only a few minutes in the emergency department; a chest x-ray was taken and interpreted at the bedside and then he was immediately "packaged" for transfer to the second floor operating suite.

Surgeon David Wisner knew that Mains was severely injured but could not know exactly how severely. "I never know until we open them up," he later told me. But, Mains was alive and on his way to surgery, and that meant he had a chance.

2

Damage Control

My memories from that month in the fall of 2001 when Jeffrey Mains became my patient are an amalgamation of drab checklists blended with vivid snapshots of blood, guts and gruesome violence. The checklists were the realm of the Trauma Nursing Unit (TNU)—where I spent every other night doing 30-hour shifts, tackling work that I would have considered simple if it were not for the overwhelming volume of it. My responsibilities were mostly drudgery but occasionally the monotony was broken by a trauma code—a "911" or "922" page[1]—that would send me sprinting to the trauma bay in the emergency department. These were moments of adrenaline, when a few minutes meant the difference and inaction could mean death.

Our trauma patients were a diverse group—the young and old, the rich and poor, the sober and drunk, the suicidal and homicidal, and the extraordinarily stupid and profoundly unlucky. Their injuries were as varied as their backgrounds—fractured arms, broken necks, bleeding spleens, leaking bowels, severed arteries, collapsed lungs, pierced hearts and much more. Rarely did I learn the patients' names; to me, they were all members of the extended Doe family with names like Ken Doe, Donald Doe, Rex Doe, Juan Doe, Cassius Doe, Dre Doe, or perhaps even John Doe.[2]

---

1. All trauma centers have alert systems of varying priority and response level. At UC Davis Medical Center, we had three trauma alerts of descending severity ("911," "922" and "933") determined by a flow sheet of criteria that included mechanism and location of injury, patient age, level of consciousness and pre-hospital vital signs (such as blood pressure). At UCDMC, the entire trauma team was only required to respond to "911" and "922" pages.
2. UCDMC, like most U.S. trauma centers, follows a well-established protocol of using made-up names for critical patients. The purpose of using fake names is to quickly establish an identity for an injured patient that facilitates rapid labeling of his or her laboratory and radiographic studies and to minimize confusion when dealing with multiple victims. Sometimes, critically injured patients may not be definitively identified for days or even weeks.

During a "911" or "922" trauma resuscitation, as others assessed the A (Airway), B (Breathing) C (Circulation) and D (Disability) of trauma's A-B-C-D-E algorithm, my responsibility was "E", Exposure and I tried to ignore the nature and circumstances of the victim's injury and just focus on excelling in this role. The best way to cut off a John Doe's pants, I'd quickly discovered, was to make a short snip through the seam with my trauma shears and then grab each cut end and tear. I relished the sound of ripping denim or polyester and raced the intern who was working on the other trouser leg, striving to reach the waistline first. The belt often caused a dilemma; it wasn't easy to cut through, even with my hardy trauma shears, and the fastest method was to unbuckle it and pull it through the belt loops. But, if I attempted this, I had to be careful not to jostle the patient or I'd get a stern rebuke from the senior surgical resident. So usually, I'd wait for the other intern to stabilize the patient's hips while I tugged on the belt. In most cases, after "E" came the not nearly so-critical "F", short for Foley catheter—a rubber bladder tube. This was a thankless task that I dreaded; it didn't matter if it were a man or a woman, the prospects for embarrassment were great. Finding a women's urethral opening, hidden between the vagina and clitoris, was tricky. To make matters worse, I always had an audience and if I didn't locate the urethra quickly envisioned snickering faces around me—nurses and senior residents—who must have been wondering about my familiarity with the female anatomy. A man's urethra was easier to find, but the catheterization process was no less hazardous. It seemed to me that the tougher the guy looked, the more dramatically he reacted—some bellowed mightily, others cussed my mother and one young punk even flailed his fists at me. My final contribution to the trauma code was what we interns sarcastically called the "WB"—warm blankets. I'd hurry to the incubator in the main ER and grab three or four thin, cream-colored blankets and drape them over the exposed and catheterized patient. Then, after only a few minutes of action, I was dismissed back to the TNU to continue my cycle of overwhelming drudgery.

When I first started with the Trauma Gold team, the trauma activation patterns seemed entirely random but within a week or so, I discerned a daily injury schedule that had some predictability. Pre-dawn was usually quiet in the trauma bay; there's something about 4a.m. that quells man's destructive tendencies, and for this I was thankful. As dawn broke on a weekday morning, though, we'd begin to see the victims of the morning commute. The nurses said that on winter mornings, when the Tule fog squatted over the Central Valley and greatly reduced visibility, rear-end fender benders were as plentiful as dirt, but even in early October commuting casualties were plentiful. Fortunately, rear-end collisions are the safest type of vehicle impact, and many of these patients came in with nothing worse than a sore neck and an impending auto body bill. Mid-day patients, on the other hand, generally weren't so fortunate. These tended to be the occupational injury patients, and their wounds could be gruesome.

Sacramento is essentially a capitol town in a vast expanse of farmland, so I shouldn't have been surprised by the variety of agricultural and industrial injuries we treated. Even now, years later, certain injuries remain vivid: the farmer who rolled his tractor over his pelvis, crushing it into a half-dozen pieces; the migrant farm worker who was thrown from a ram-shackle pick-up and suffered eight broken ribs and a collapsed lung; the four man crew with severe insecticide poisoning; the young man from the quarry who had been pinned under 800 pounds of granite for three hours, and the water treatment worker who slipped and fell 30 feet into a concrete tank, breaking both femurs before collapsing into sewage.

The late afternoon's business was no more palatable because this was when the injured children arrived. Despite what many parents (and the media) may think, school is a pretty safe place. It's after-school that's dangerous. Bike accidents, falls from the monkey bars, failures to look both ways before crossing the street, and (this was always heart wrenching) toddlers mistakenly backed over by a parent's vehicle in the driveway; kids were magnets for mishaps after the final bell rang.

Supper time brought an occasional reprieve. I attributed this to the fact that evening was the hottest time of day in the Central Valley. For those who haven't had occasion to experience it firsthand, I can unequivocally attest that Sacramento is positively broiling in the summer months. Not the heavy, thick-with-moisture heat of the East Coast, but an equally oppressive scalding desert heat, the type that might melt your leather car seat, or as in my minivan's case, cause your rear-view mirror to come unglued and drop off the windshield. On the hottest of summer days, when ultraviolet light seemed to bore into my skull, paralyzing temperatures would peak around 6p.m. That June, we had an early heat wave with a long series of 100-plus-degree days. California was facing an energy crisis, and there were dire predictions of widespread brownouts. Ads saturated the airwaves imploring residents to "Flex their Power" by setting the thermostat at 78 degrees and to be aware of unnecessary lights and other "Watts going on." Fortunately, the relative lack of humidity allowed for a nightly respite, and as soon as the sun set, we could open our windows and let the crisp air permeate the house. But as the city woke up in the cool night, the hospital became once again inundated with a potpourri of traumatic injuries, many of which were the result of high speed motor vehicle collisions.

I grew up two hours west of Sacramento in affluent Marin County and as a kid, I viewed Sacramento as a place that one traveled *through* (on the way to the mountains) rather than *to*. Viewed from Interstate 80, stumpy "skyscrapers" rise disjointedly over bland terrain and fail to inspire visions of a big city. Only the confluence of two rivers, the American and Sacramento, adds a touch of place, an explanation for this accumulation of roads, homes, and telephone poles. An infamous bridge, painted a strange sickly shade of gold, spans the Sacramento River near downtown and is visible from I-80—but I found it far less worthy of rubbernecking than its neighboring Coors Light billboard which, that fall, celebrated "Raider Nation" with the well-contoured midriff of a cheerleader. After I officially moved to Sacramento, I discovered that my boyhood perception of the city was more or less spot on.

More than anything, Sacramento *is* a city that people drive through. Within its limits, two vast interstates intersect—I-80, which runs from the Atlantic to the Pacific, and I-5 which runs from Mexico to Canada and at all hours, a steady stream of autos flows through the city, heading east, west, north and south. At the UCDMC, we saw the human carnage of their collisions. Compounding the challenge of managing the large volume of local car crashes was the influx of patients transported from afar. Because UCDMC is the only Level I trauma center[3] in central California for hundreds of miles in every direction, critically injured patients were often helicoptered in from remote places, little rural towns with names like Galt, Cool, Weed, and Red Bluff. Many of the people injured in these obscure locales and transported to see us were victims of thrill-seeking endeavors gone awry—snowboarders with broken legs, people beat up from the feet up after being thrown from their all-terrain vehicles, and riders ejected from their horses. I recall one particularly gory calamity from the Sacramento River Delta—a water-skier whose arm got caught in the tow line and suffered what is called a degloving injury. The force of the taut line accelerating against the arm of the falling skier caused his skin and muscle to be pulled completely off, like a glove, leaving behind nothing but bone and tendon.

Later in the night, the shootings and stabbings began. Sacramento may be surrounded by farms, but it has big city crime with a multicultural flavor. I was initially surprised to learn that Sacramento is the most ethnically diverse metropolitan area in the U.S., but several nights in our trauma bay satisfied my

---

3.   The highest of four levels of trauma designation bestowed on hospitals by the American College of Surgeons.

doubts.[4] We saw all different types of people shooting and stabbing each other, some in gangs, some not: Aryans like Joseph Ferguson, former Soviet state immigrants like Nikolay Soltys, Hispanics, Laotians, Vietnamese, Pacific Islanders, African-Americans, and just about any other color or ethnicity you could think of.

I estimated that about 90 percent of our late night visitors were intoxicated in some way. Alcohol, cocaine, heroin, GHB, ecstasy, PCP, and methamphetamine—lots of methamphetamine (also known as meth, crank, or crystal). With time, it became easy for me to identify those flying on meth—their "accidents" always had a similar flavor, a combination of bizarre, stupid, and destructive acts.[5] There was, for instance, the contractor who had nail-gunned his hand to a 2x4 while working in his poorly lit garage in the middle of the night and the woman with several cracked vertebrae who refused to lie still and shouted at me, "Yeah I'm on crank … but this is nothing … I can crank harder than this." Some time later, I saw an article about a Portland-area man who, while high on methamphetamine, had shot 12 nails, each up to two inches in length, into his skull and somehow survived without significant injury. Unfortunately, self-inflicted wounds like this often appeared at 3a.m., just as I was lying down for an hour of precious sleep: ice pick wound to the abdomen, steak knife to the heart, or razor blade to the wrists.

From around 10p.m. to 3a.m. on the weekend nights I spent most of my time in the trauma bay, leaving only briefly to retrieve warm blankets for the injured, drunk, and suicidal. I'd then return to the TNU to prepare for my morning rounds. Often, I was so numbed by fatigue and work that the horror of what I'd just witnessed wouldn't register for days, sometimes not until my wife looked at me sadly and asked "did that really happen?" When I returned home from a shift on the trauma service I was zombie-like—plodding around the house without purpose or slumped on the couch and utterly incapable of communicating in full sentences or engaging in the simplest decision-making such as what to watch on TV. It wasn't until weeks or months later that I realized how the consequences of the violence that I saw permanently altered my relationship with risk. Despite my

---

4.   Based on a Harvard study of 2000 census data published in *Time Magazine*.

5.   Methamphetamine addicts can also be easily identified by the presence of "Meth Mouth." A combination of the drug's high acidity, its tendency to cause teeth grinding and trigger cravings for high-calorie carbonated beverages and its long duration of action have devastating effects on teeth. An addict with full blown "Meth Mouth" has stained, rotting and shrunken teeth (as if filed down for a dental crown) that often can be spotted from across the room.

wife's repeated urging, I continue to refuse her invitations to join her for a romantic horseback ride on the beach—I don't think I could find it romantic—not with the memory of the 17-year-old girl who I'd seen die in front of me from a massive head injury after being thrown from a horse. Likewise, I will never knowingly live close to anyone with pit bulls—not after seeing what such dogs did to a poor 7-year-old boy—grotesquely tearing and puncturing his body until it became a corpse. At one time, in my adventurous years, I might have thought it exhilarating to jump out of an airplane, but any desire to do so was snuffed when I saw two young parachuters dead-on-arrival because of an equipment malfunction.

My most lasting trauma bay memories were spawned from the gory and the tragic, but there is one patient that I remember because of his creativity and his persistence. His name was Donald and he was a carpenter, an epileptic carpenter, with a penchant for falling from great heights. Or, I should say, pretending to fall from great heights. I never learned Donald's exact age—he looked to be in his late 30's but could have been much younger—but my colleagues made sure that I knew about his past. Years ago, he had undergone major cranial surgery to remove a large seizure-inducing AVM (arteriovenous malformation) and the operation left him with a large, depressed defect in his blockish skull. At some point during his complicated recovery, Donald became hooked on an assortment of pain-killers and sedatives and, to make matters worse, his seizures persisted. At least that's what he led everyone to believe. He would often come to the ED and fake a seizure in the waiting room so that he could get a fix of his favorite drugs. When the triage nurses got hip to this act, Donald changed his tack and figured out how to arrive in the ED as a "911" trauma code. The details were a little different each time, but the essence of his tale was pretty much the same; he'd suffered a seizure, fallen and hit his head. Maybe it was while he was on a roof or on a ladder or while working on gutters or while riding his bike. Oddly, there were never any witnesses and it was never exactly clear who had called for help. When the paramedics arrived and heard Donald's account and noticed his misshapen skull (and Donald always made sure they noticed) they were alarmed—someone who hadn't seen Donald before could easily mistake his misshapen noggin for an acute depressed skull fracture. He'd be rushed in, Code 3, with the whole trauma team waiting in the trauma bay for the "head injury patient status post seizure." The first half-dozen or so times he staged this, Donald received the whole battery of tests—x-rays, CT of the head and abdomen, and a full rainbow of lab tests. Everything always came up negative (except the tax payers' bottom line, because guess who picked up the bill?) and by the time it had, Donald was drugged, happy, and ready to go. Eventually, the response to Donald's cries of "wolf" became less urgent and the senior ED or trauma resident would intervene before a full trauma code was activated. Whenever a paramedic report contained the phrases "depressed," "skull fracture," "seizures," and "fall," someone was dispatched to meet Donald at the door, and if no new injuries were seen, to downgrade the trauma. Donald, once he realized that he would be made to wait, like all the other non-critically injured patients, would usually pull off his cervical collar, curse, and stomp out of the ED, only to try the whole stunt again a few days later.

On any given day, I had no idea how many critical traumas or new admissions I would have. This, combined with all of my other errands, suppressed my curiosity and drove me to maximize efficiency. In order to round on 30 patients each day, attend every trauma code and perhaps catch a meal or two, I had to be supremely efficient. So, I used every spare moment not spent gulping down a grease-saturated specialty from the cafeteria to prepare my notes for the next day. I kept 30 some pieces of blue-trimmed progress note paper stuffed in my long white coat, along with a collection of pocket medical reviews, laminated reference cards and my green trauma shears. Scrawled on each piece of note paper were the patient's name, medical record number, and the outline of the "SOAP" note I was writing. The first time, as a third-year medical student, that I was asked to write a "SOAP" note, I was confused. I knew how to write a daily progress note, a brief recap of the past day's events, current vital signs and physical exam. But what was a "SOAP" note? A cleansing of the medical record? Some type of cover up for negligent care? No, it turned out that "SOAP" didn't stand for anything that interesting, but instead for the four elements of a proper daily progress note: *S*ubjective, *O*bjective, *A*ssessment and *P*lan. Virtually all medical specialties that treat inpatients utilize the SOAP note, but while the practice is widespread, its execution can vary greatly. A SOAP note on the medicine service may be a several page document including a long list of medications, lab results, and an updated list of possible diagnoses. On the psychiatry service it might be heavily waited towards the *S*ubjective—with a detailed description, for example, of a patient's belief that a monkey is lighting bottle rockets in the bathroom. On surgical services, SOAP notes were expected to be brief, unadorned and devoid of interpretation. Consider the SOAP note I wrote on Jeffrey Mains for October 20th, 2001 [with translations of abbreviations].

S: Tolerating small amounts of p.o. [by mouth]. Ambulating with difficulty. Requiring decreased pain meds. "Restless" + Flatus [gas] + eating bread OK. No N/V [nausea or vomiting]

O: Vitals: AVSS [Afebrile, Vital Signs Stable]
Resp: Lungs CTA B/L [lungs clear to auscultation bilaterally]
CV: RRR, no m, r, g [Regular rate and rhythm. No murmurs, rubs or gallops]
Abd: Soft, NT [non-tender]. Wound dressing c/d/i [clean, dry and intact]
A/P: 27 yo male with GSW [gunshot wound] to abdomen with enterocu-
taneous fistula. Day 14/14 of antibiotics. Continue to advance diet as tolerated.
Continue TPN [intravenous nutrition] as needed. Continue ambulate.
Continue IS [incentive spirometry][6]

I found this note in his medical record, and when I re-read it was reminded of
how I rushed to prepare this and other progress notes; of how I scribbled while
standing next to the radiologist or while on the phone with a nurse. And I was
not surprised that the brevity of this October 20th SOAP note belied the progress
that Jeffrey Mains had made since the night he'd nearly died. As I later found,
this story too had much more to it.

◆   ◆   ◆

Trauma surgeons often refer to the peritoneal cavity as having "potential."
This is not a flattering description. It doesn't mean that the peritoneal cavity, like
a rookie centerfielder, has the "potential" for greatness. Instead, it is an anatomical distinction, a potential space between organs. The peritoneum is a thin mem-
branous layer that surrounds the stomach, intestines, and other abdominal organs
and their blood supply. It has two components, a visceral layer and parietal layer
and the space in between is the peritoneal cavity. Because the intestines tend to
expand and retract with the passage of food, the peritoneum is a stretchy covering, able to handle either Weight Watchers or Thanksgiving dinner. Normally,
the peritoneal cavity is small, filled with only a tea cup's worth of lubricating
fluid, but it can accommodate much more. In the case of a traumatic injury,
blood may leak or pour into the peritoneal cavity, and if the bleeding isn't controlled expediently, shock and death can quickly follow. Jeffrey Mains was young
and his heart was healthy, so he was able to temporarily compensate for the loss
of blood into his peritoneal cavity. But, even the healthiest of hearts cannot work
without blood. Like an engine when it runs out of its gas, a heart without blood
will stall.

---

6.   This is a simple breathing machine that encourages patients to take deep breaths and
fully expand their lungs.

In the early morning of September 10ᵗʰ, 2001, Jeffrey Mains was wheeled into a second floor operating room. He was put under general anesthesia, given a breathing tube, and connected to a ventilator. Dr. Wisner, with assistance from his senior resident, Jeremy Benedetti, performed an exploratory laparotomy. The surgeons made a scalpel incision from just below the breastbone (sternum) to just above the bladder and incised and retracted the underlying tissue and then entered the peritoneum. Inside was a bloody mess. Wisner and Benedetti packed the entire abdomen with dry sponges to soak up the hemorrhage and then explored for sources of bleeding. The spleen appeared clean, uninjured. The liver had a large laceration which was re-packed with sponges until the bleeding was controlled. There was a hole in the right hemi-diaphragm and a palpable bullet fragment in the superficial right chest that was removed and held for the police as evidence. Then the surgeons "ran" the bowel, segment by segment searching for injury. The gut was bruised and bleeding from multiple sites and completely sev-ered midway through the small bowel in the area of the jejunum. Sections of the large bowel, in the right colon and transverse colon, were also injured and dying. The dying and dead bowel tissue was removed and the interposing ends stapled, leaving Mains with a dead end gut, like a road barricaded at multiple locations. As the operation progressed, the patient's temperature dipped lower and the operative report notes that there was "increased ooze throughout the abdomen." Mains was progressing from shock to coagulopathy—a diffuse thinning of the blood—a common complication of traumatic injury.

Dr. Wisner decided to cease further repair and exploration and attempt to sta-bilize his patient with medication to coagulate the blood. It was three in the morning and he was not optimistic. In the waiting room outside the operating room he met with Jeffrey's mother, Linda, and uncle, Gary Kambestad. Hours earlier, Linda Mains had fallen asleep while watching the late news. Before she nodded off she noted that the lead story was on a series of nearby shootings and for a moment she worried about Jeffrey, but then thought, "He has to be at work early tomorrow. He's at home and safe." At 2a.m., she learned that Jeffrey was actually not home and not at all safe.

"Dr. Wisner told us that Jeff wasn't going to make it, that he had bled out," Linda Mains recalled, years later. "He told us that he was still alive but that it was going to be a long day and that we should go home, shower, and notify the fam-ily."

On the morning of September 11ᵗʰ, 2001, Jeffrey Mains, to the surprise of his nurses, family and doctors, was still alive. Despite being in very critical condition, Mains returned to the operating room. His first surgery had been "damage control," this one was clean-up. Liver packs were removed, sections of bowel reattached to one another with sutures and the entire abdomen re-explored.

Mains woke up on September 12th in the SICU, the Surgical Intensive Care Unit. He was confused and delirious and the TV in his room didn't help—on it a video of a passenger plane flying into a tall building was being played over and over. "I was so drugged up," Mains later told me, "that I didn't know what was up or down, but I was hearing people and voices on the TV." The atmosphere in the SICU and throughout the hospital was tense. Health care professionals attempted to continue their work and maintain their composure despite the shock of the terrorist attacks and the uncertainty of what the next target might be. When Linda Mains arrived at the SICU to visit her son, she saw nurses crowded around a TV in the waiting room, watching the news. "And I thought, 'My god, all of those people will never get to see their families again.' To be honest, I almost felt a little grateful about my situation." For Jeffrey Mains, on the other hand, the circumstances were too much. Beset by agitation and panic, he thrashed on his gurney and on September 13th, loosened his hands from his restraints and pulled out his breathing tube. After that, he was kept deeply sedated for days. Visitors came and went hourly, his mother and uncle were there every day and his sister visited frequently. High school friends, friends from the police force, ex-girlfriends, and a current girlfriend, the one who wanted a long term commitment (but whom Linda Mains wanted to just go away) shuffled in and out of the SICU. Even Jeffrey's father visited once, but when Mains' heart rate tripled under the aura of his father's words, his dad was asked to leave. The recovery, if there was to be a recovery, would be very slow.

3

Remember the Tiger

By the end of one month as an intern on the Trauma Gold team, perspective had become a deism-like entity; I knew it was out there but I wasn't sure where or in what form. Immersed as I'd been in my cycle of efficiency punctuated occasionally with a sprint to the ED, I hadn't had much of an opportunity to consider the "why" of what I'd been doing. For example, I was well-versed in the specifics of the primary survey (the A-B-C-D-E algorithm) but I had no idea who had first described it or how long it had been in use. Also, I'd grasped the basic structure of Sacramento's regional trauma system but I didn't realize how nascent the coordinated care of traumatic injury actually was. If I'd done my residency training elsewhere, any glimpse of perspective may have indefinitely escaped me, but I was at UCDMC, home to Dr. William Blaisdell. I never met Dr. Blaisdell during my three years of residency—he'd retired from clinical practice some years before—but his legend was nevertheless inescapable. He was, I was repeatedly told in hushed reverence, one of the founding fathers of modern trauma care. Of course, it wasn't until after residency that I had a holistic appreciation of what this meant.

In the mid-1960's, when William Blaisdell became the chief of surgery at San Francisco General Hospital, coordinated responses to traumatic injury existed nowhere but on the battlefield. Back then, a gunshot victim such as Jeffrey Mains would have been treated much differently. A bystander calling for help wouldn't have dialed 9-1-1, for that service didn't exist. Instead, he or she would have needed to thumb through the White pages to find help. Emergency phone numbers existed, but residents needed to consult the front of their phonebooks to find them and there was great regional variability. For example, in the eight counties of 1970's era Kansas City, there were 78 different emergency phone numbers for 45 different ambulance companies. Even if someone had figured out how to call for help, a victim such as Mains wouldn't have had access to a fully-equipped ambulance or paramedic team and if he received transport at all, it would likely have been in a hearse, driven by one of the approximately 12,000 undertakers who supplemented their incomes by using their vehicles, sometimes converted for medical use, sometimes not, as transport for injured patients. During the ride, he wouldn't have received any treatment because most "ambulance" morticians worked alone and had no training in first aid. There would have been no radio contact[1] between the undertaker and the trauma center either, and actually, no trauma center at all. Had Mains made it to an emergency department, he would have been treated by physicians with little or no training in the care of penetrating trauma and limited resuscitative resources. In this era, most of the doctors staffing emergency departments were not trained in emergency medicine and were interns or residents—early in their training for other specialties and working 24- or even 48-hour shifts. Jeffrey Mains would have, most certainly, died an unnecessary death. And in this respect he would have had ample company.

Today, we know that about half of all traumatic deaths occur within minutes of injury. Most of these victims perish from massive hemorrhage (uncontrolled bleeding) or severe nervous system interruption. These types of injuries are untreatable—there is no meaningful therapy for a spinal cord pulverized by the high speed collision of a head into pavement or an aorta ripped in two by the force of abrupt deceleration. The remaining half of traumatic fatalities occur minutes to weeks later and can have a myriad of causes, including delayed bleeding, neurological dysfunction, infection, blood clots, and organ failure. Many of these sub-acute deaths can be prevented if injuries are recognized and treated in an expedited manner. Even in the 1960's, Dr. Blaisdell and his contemporaries knew this. In 1965 alone, 107,000 Americans died from accidental injuries (49,000 in motor vehicle crashes) and trauma was the leading cause of death for those between the ages of 1 and 37.[2] The available evidence suggested that many of these deaths were preventable. For example, a 1961 survey of 782 traffic deaths in California found that accidents occurring in rural counties were almost four

---

1.   Communication between rescue vehicles and emergency departments was about as standard as cruise control on a Model T. "Although it is possible to converse with astronauts in outer space," noted the National Academy of Sciences in 1966, "communication is seldom possible between an ambulance and the emergency department it is approaching."

2.   The resulting cost to the public in medical expenses, property damage, lost wages and administrative costs was almost $18 billion. In today's era of inflated spending ($18 billion gets you a snazzy fighter plane or two) this sum may seem trivial, but at the time it was nearly equal to the government's annual appropriation for the Vietnam War.

times more likely to be fatal than those in urban areas and that rural victims had significantly longer transport times and died of less serious injuries. Other studies, based on autopsy reports of highway fatalities, reported that up to 25% of the deaths were either definitely or possibly preventable. In some instances, the transport of accident victims was morosely backwards—in a highly publicized incident in Los Angeles County, morticians responded to a multi-casualty vehicle accident by first transporting the *dead*, and then returning for the injured. Even those who received rapid transport to medical facilities or arrived in salvageable condition had a poor prognosis. A review of seriously injured soldiers treated at civilian hospitals between 1957 and 1960 demonstrated that 1 out of 6 died from potentially treatable conditions. The tragic irony for these soldiers was that they would have had better outcomes if they'd received their medical care from the military. Three major armed conflicts in the first part of the 20th-century had taught the military a great deal about treating traumatic injury and death rates among battle casualties had declined significantly with each conflict: 8% in World War I, 4.5% in World War II and 2.5% in the Korean War. By 1966, military expertise was such that the National Academy of Sciences, in its landmark report *Accidental Death and Disability: the Neglected Disease of Modern Society*, stated that "if seriously wounded, the chances of survival would be better in the zone of combat than on the average city street."

For William Blasidell, I later discovered, the impetus for change began in a different war zone, the Haight-Ashbury. In the mid-1960's, as the anti-war movement and counter-culture burgeoned in San Francisco, so did drugs, and with drugs, drug-related violence. As Chief of Surgery at San Francisco General Hospital (SFGH), Blaisdell's job included managing care in the ED and beginning in 1966, he detected a dramatic increase in the violent byproducts of LSD and PCP-fertilized "flower power." Between 1966 and 1968, the number of victims of violent crime treated at San Francisco General quadrupled and by 1969 the rate of penetrating trauma was sevenfold greater than it had been ten years before. With thousands of youths tripping on psychedelic substances, the inevitable daily assortment of bad trips further strained available emergency and psychiatric care. Blaisdell's emergency department, which was staffed primarily by surgical residents, was inefficient and overwhelmed. In his historical account, *Catastrophes, Epidemics and Neglected Diseases*, Blaisdell recounts an illustrative case: a patient complaining of back pain "was asked to sit on the bench and wait his turn, until the woman he sat next to screamed and pointed to a knife sticking in his back." Driven by the necessity to improve care for such patients, Blaisdell set about implementing the country's first city-wide trauma program. Towards this end, he was aided by the fact that San Francisco already had a single ED dedicated to receiving ambulance patients (San Francisco General's Mission Emergency) as well as one of the best ambulance systems in existence. Whereas much of the nation was served by ill-equipped hearses without much in the way of communication or treatment capabilities, San Francisco had a fleet of ambulances with prescient features—such as two-way radios, airway modalities and room for multiple casualties—and were staffed by "stewards" who were capable of administering basic stabilization measures. Blaisdell coordinated with these ambulances to standardize the pre-hospital response and created a dedicated "trauma team" to accept and manage patients. The squad consisted of an ED team staffed in 12 hours shifts by two interns and one resident who exclusively treated trauma victims and two ward (inpatient) teams with two interns and one resident each. The teams were supervised by a chief (6th year) resident who was on service (and lived in the hospital) for two months at a time, and a rotating attending. In an era when residents in other specialties, according to Blaisdell's recollection, arrived to work in "sandals, tie died T-shirts, and work pants," sporting "long hair, beards and mustaches and love beads" and "judging from body odor [having] neglected to bathe," these surgical residents were required to wear conventional white uniforms and maintain cleanliness. This dress code was emblematic of Blaisdell's attempt to institute a highly organized and militaristic approach to trauma care. And in short order, he succeeded—in 1968 the San Francisco General Trauma Center was established with the goal of providing "immediate resuscitation and definitive treatment for all victims of injury." The San Francisco model helped to spur others[3] to coordinate response to traumatic injury and in 1972 SFGH became one of the first nine federally funded trauma centers in the United States.

A decade after establishing a trauma center in San Francisco, Blaisdell traveled 120 miles east to assume control of the trauma program at a hospital (Sacramento General) that would soon become UC Davis Medical Center. From that day on, trauma care in Sacramento was done one way, and one way only, the Blaisdell way. For the most part, Blaisdell followed established trauma protocols such as Advanced Trauma Life Support (ATLS). He had, after all, helped to develop them. There were, however, certain idiosyncrasies, one of which I witnessed on the first day of my trauma internship. I recall standing in the back of the trauma bay having arrived a minute later than the patient and feeling completely useless. Two other interns had already brandished their trauma shears and were at work

---

3.   Several other pioneers deserve mention here: R Adams Cowley in Maryland, David Boyd in Chicago and Blaisdell's protégé, Donald Trunkey.

on denim pant legs. A somewhat tentative junior resident with a prominent hook nose was assessing the A-B-C's and had just reported the blood pressure and moved on to D (Disability) when his senior barked at him "check the belly." The junior looked up with submissive confusion and then complied—pressing on the patient's rotund midsection several times before declaring "abdomen soft and non-tender." I too was confused, for I'd dutifully studied the ATLS guidelines and was pretty certain that an abdominal exam was not part of the A-B-C's but rather of the secondary survey that followed them. This may not seem like a significant difference, but remember that trauma resuscitations nowadays are extremely regimented and deviations from the protocols are not usually tolerated. The ED attending must have noticed my questioning gaze. He leaned over to me and said, "That's how Blaisdell always wanted it done." Then he added "Blaisdell loved the abdomen, loved it."

Indeed, it was true. Dr. Blaisdell had exhibited a long-standing passion for the abdominal exam and believed that it should not necessarily be restricted to superficial means. "Laparotomy [surgical exploration of the abdomen] is the natural extension of the abdominal exam," was a famed Blaisdell justification for rushing a trauma patient to the operating room. High resolution CT scans had given Blaisdell's disciples another diagnostic tool that could be used in lieu of surgery to evaluate patients with suspected abdominal injuries, yet they continued to respect Blaisdell's deviation in the primary survey. And as the intern in charge of Foley catheters and warm blankets, I concluded that it was not my place to point out the discrepancy. Nor did I ever assail the necessity of including a manual rectal exam with every trauma's secondary survey. Fortunately for me, this job belonged to the second year resident, but yet I still often winced at the uniformity with which it was administered—even to patients who had isolated or superficial-appearing injuries. Out of earshot, we referred to this intrusion as the "UC Davis handshake" and it was sometimes unannounced, or even worse, announced incorrectly (I once overheard a resident tell a patient, "Sir now you are going to feel *your* finger in *my* bottom.)" The battery of trauma laboratory tests, called a rainbow because it utilized every possible color of collection tube, performed on virtually every trauma patient also puzzled me. Was it really necessary, I wondered, to check clotting studies in healthy young people or obtain an alcohol level in an eight year-old boy? Not everything we did made sense to me but, like the other interns, I trusted the prevailing wisdom of Dr. Blaisdell and his disciples. Eventually, it dawned on me that their treatment protocols were designed to limit the critical thinking of the young doctors who implemented them. If things were done the same way, every time, nothing would be missed. If selective judgment was used, in particular selective *intern* judgment, something might be over-looked. For awhile, this presumption that I was not to be trusted to make clinical decisions irritated me, but this was because I was looking at it from an individual-istic, rather than a systems viewpoint. In reality, there was no need for me to make clinical decisions when well-established protocols could make them for me. In those situations in which the protocols didn't have the answer, we turned to Dr. Wisner.

The surgical residents referred to Dr. David Wisner as "The Wiz"; a tribute to the breakneck speed at which he conducted morning rounds. Like the others, I was impressed by his ability to make rapid clinical assessments and decisions, but was even more impressed with the quiet authority he exuded. Surgeons are often portrayed as brilliant but volatile characters—always on the edge of ripping into a subordinate who isn't getting it quite right. Not Wisner, his voice was soft and reserved yet somehow carried a hundred decibels worth of strength. His physical presence was undeniable, he was as stout as ironwood, but there was something more. During many trauma resuscitations he would stand silently in the back of the trauma bay, letting the fellow or senior resident run the show and occasion-ally providing guidance with gentle queries. As soon as a resuscitation went off track or became chaotic, however, he took over. "Ok everybody, I am running this code," he'd firmly declare. "Anyone who is not doing anything here needs to leave this room." Whenever he did this, and the huddle of gawkers dissipated, it set me at ease. No matter how sick our patient appeared, Wisner had the situa-tion under control. I have no doubt that Wisner's mentor, William Blaisdell, had in his day demonstrated a similar aura of calm leadership.

Although Wisner had been chief for some time, he still honored many of his mentor's traditions. Like Blaisdell, he often jogged the stairs during morning rounds, sometimes up seven flights straight, a ritual that occasionally (and one might say predictably) caused a sleep deprived resident to pass out. The two trauma services, the Blue and Gold, were named after the two separate surgical services Blaisdell had established at San Francisco General in 1968. Wisner's Socratic teaching style was straight from the Blaisdell playbook, and while this rarely surfaced while we whizzed through rounds on the (mostly uncomplicated) TNU patients, it was clearly evident in other forums, such as his lectures to resi-dents and students. Wisner also continued the Blaisdell practice of using fictional situations to teach important surgical principles. The story I recall best is that of the tiger.

"That was classic Blaisdell," Wisner later explained to me. "He would start out by asking all of us, as he peered through his black horn-rim glasses 'Why is it dangerous to shoot a tiger?' Those who hadn't heard the story before would fumble and stammer, trying to answer, not having any idea what he was talking about. The answer was that if you shot a tiger, a muscular tiger with layers of tawny flesh rippling under its fur, you couldn't track it because it wouldn't bleed. The overlying fur and skin would cover up the wound and that tiger might be bleeding internally, but you would have no way of knowing unless you captured him or he died. Blaisdell would have us all going, picturing ourselves hunting down a tiger in an Asian jungle. Maybe the tiger's hurt, maybe not. And when you weren't looking, the tiger would jump from a branch and eat you. Then he'd look at us sternly and tell us to always remember that in a trauma you couldn't tell by the wounds on the outside what was hurt on the inside ... Remember the tiger."

Thinking back to the day that Jeffrey Mains was discharged from the Trauma Nursing Unit, I am reminded of Blaisdell's proverb. By then, Mains' external wounds had mostly healed over and, scarred as he was, it was impossible to tell from the outside the extent to which he was hurt on the inside.

♦   ♦   ♦

For 23 days, Jeffrey Mains had been a resident of the second floor SICU and he'd remained in critical condition throughout. Wisner repeatedly told Jeffrey's mother, Linda Mains, that he was not optimistic that her son would recover. "I don't think he ever really gave up on Jeffrey," said Linda Mains, "but he didn't want us to expect too much. It was like that for twenty days." On September 17th, Mains returned to the operating room for re-exploration and to have multiple abscesses drained. He was back in the OR on September 27th to have the fluid collecting in his lung removed by a procedure called VATS (video assisted thoracic surgery). Afterwards, Mains developed an enterocutaneous fistula—a communicating tunnel between his bowel and skin that meant feces came out in the wrong place. He was on multiple antibiotics, multiple pain medications, received his nutrition through IV fluids and hadn't had a normal bowel movement for over two weeks. Although now awake and alert, Mains still had difficulty speaking because of residual tracheal swelling from where the breathing tube had been and was unable to use his (dominant) left arm because of a painful blood clot. Understandably frustrated, he barely even attempted to communicate.

Even as preparations were made to downgrade Mains' care to the Trauma Nursing unit (TNU), an ominous cloud seemed to hover over him. But on that 23rd day in the SICU, that cloud thinned as four words were scrawled on a piece of plain white paper. With an unsteady right hand, Mains wrote a simple message to his family, "We will make it." For Linda Mains this was the point where cautious optimism turned to belief, belief that her son would someday go home and that the essence of his character was intact. "Jeffrey is such a gentle person," she later told me "and he never wants to impose on others. It wasn't about him, it was about us. He didn't write 'I will make it,' no it was 'We will make it.'"

But Mains' recovery wasn't as simple as four scribbled words, in fact things would get worse before they got better. For days after being transferred to the TNU, Mains slouched on his bed, looking gaunt and defeated. His pain was difficult to control and he didn't want to walk, in fact he could barely stand because of the tension from his abdominal scars and he had to be coaxed to take sips of fluid. His blood tests were still abnormal; he was anemic and his body's white blood cell count was double the normal value, indicating that he was still fighting off infection despite being on two strong IV antibiotics. Slowly though, spurred by his family's encouragement, he progressed. A physical therapist forced him to get up and move, teaching him, step by step, how to walk again. One evening he was brought a large tray of food—lasagna, salad, and more—laid out on a tablecloth in front of his hospital bed. He kept the meal down, but it didn't stay in his system for long. "It was like my innards were brand new," he later recalled. Over the next few days, supplemented by a steady diet of Jamba Juice smoothies, those remodeled innards began to function again.

The psychological improvement was less steady and Mains had frequent episodes of acute anxiety. He repeatedly re-lived the moments before and after the shooting ... pulling up to the stoplight in his truck, the commotion, the sound of shots ripping through metal. The realization that he'd been shot. Stepping out on to the road. Collapsing. Conscious one moment, blackness the next. Restrained and groggy in a strange room with beeping lights and pictures of planes flying into buildings on the TV. Twenty-three days in the SICU.

Mains saw a psychiatrist, who on October 18th, wrote the following: "Mood anxious with tearful affect. He has felt very sad and anxious, cries all the time, can't sleep more than three hours at night; has recurrent thoughts about the shooting, is hyper vigilant [heightened awareness of surroundings] and jumpy. Also, feels depressed to the point of not wanting to do anything." Based on these observations, Mains was diagnosed with acute stress disorder and started on a trial of Valium.

"It was the saddest time," said Linda Mains. "It was always sad, but now he was cognizant of the pain, and of the situation. It was a tough time in that trauma unit." Mains no longer had a room and a nurse to himself and he saw less of Dr. Wisner and more of inexperienced interns like me. And as he began to eat and walk again, it got worse. His mom remembers him as "Constantly sobbing," and "just unable to pull it together." He was also becoming angry, and no one blamed him. Chance had played him a wicked game, put him in the path of a maniac with an arsenal of weapons and he had the right to be pissed off about that. "How did that kid get a weapon like that?" he once asked me. "An AK-47, an automatic assault rifle. In the middle of Sacramento, just shooting people ..." Everyone agreed that it was time for Jeffrey to go home; surely the emotional recovery would be faster there because it was going backward in the TNU. On October 24th, we removed the last remaining intra-abdominal drain, took out the IV, packaged up some dressing supplies for the remaining open abdominal wounds, prescribed over 100 pain pills, and sent Jeffrey Mains home.

4

Own the Airway

In September 2003, two years after Joseph Ferguson shot and nearly killed Jeffrey Mains, I found myself once again immersed in the A-B-C's of trauma resuscitation. The difference was that, two years later and in my first month as a senior resident, I was in charge of "A," and this meant I was expected to own the airway. When I first heard this phrase, "own the airway," I thought it presumptuous—how could a physician "own" a patient's airway as if it was a commodity? Surely, a person's trachea was more innately his or her own than a moped or a surfboard? With time, however, I came to appreciate the phrase because it captured the mentality necessary to learn a critical skill. Training in emergency medicine emphasizes, above all else, the skill of airway management and with good reason; when a patient ceases to breathe immediate action is required. Bodily organs deprived of oxygen fare poorly and basic functions, such as the heartbeat, rapidly lose their verve. Depending on factors such as patient age and health, there might be minutes to spare, or maybe only seconds.

As the senior resident in charge of "A", I had to be ready, on a moment's notice, to control the airway of a patient who could no longer breathe for himself. In these critical situations, I could begin with temporizing techniques such as medications, oxygen and breathing masks. But if these didn't work or the patient couldn't adequately protect his airway,[1] he needed a breathing tube and a ventilator. The process of inserting a breathing tube, called intubation, fills even a seasoned emergency physician with trepidation. This is because while intubations are usually straightforward, they can also be very challenging and if things go wrong, they can go very wrong. During the first two years of my residency, I'd studied the procedure in texts, practiced on a mannequin named Dorothy and performed it on a few actual patients, always in controlled settings. I'd thor-

---

1. Unconscious or intoxicated patients cannot "protect" their airways if they have lost the ability to gag (the gag reflex). These patients are at high risk of choking on (aspirating) their own vomit.

oughly memorized and re-memorized the sequence for the emergent intubation using a pneumonic called the "6 P's": 1) *pre*-oxygenate, 2) *p*repare suction, 3) *p*osition (the patient's head) properly 4) *p*re-medicate (with paralyzing and sedating medications), 5) *p*ush paralyzing medications and 6) *p*rotect the airway (by holding pressure over the neck to prevent aspiration).

I visualized the technique frequently—while jogging, sitting through a dull lecture, cruising in my minivan on I-80, or watching a romantic comedy with my wife. I hoped that with enough visualization, the procedure would feel natural when I needed to perform it for real. The snapshots in my imagination were consistent; open the patient's mouth using an exaggerated right thumb and forefinger snap; grasp the L-shaped laryngoscope with my left hand and introduce it into the mouth at an angle; slide the blade to the left side of the tongue and push the tongue slightly up and away; pop the curved tip of the blade into the valleculla, the small space between the tongue and the epiglottis; using my shoulder as a fulcrum, firmly push up and out; wait for the vocal cords, an ellipse of raised white outlining a dark tunnel, to pop into view; keep my eye trained on the cords while an assistant handed me the endotracheal tube, a clear plastic tube fitted with a metal stylet and with a slight hockey-stick curve at its end; with my right hand, slowly guide the tube over the tongue and advance several centimeters into the dark tunnel; maintain grip on the tube while withdrawing the laryngoscope blade and removing the metal stylet; inflate the endotracheal tube's balloon with 10cc of air and check for proper placement; look for the comforting sight of mist in the tube; listen for breath sounds in both lungs and place and check the color change detector; yellow was good; purple was bad.

Before my 3rd year of residency, I'd physically performed this sequence enough that it sometimes felt as smooth and rehearsed in actuality as it was in fantasy. Other times it felt as smooth as a mountain bike's tire tread, or as full of hiccups as driving a manual transmission car for the first time. I'd cracked a tooth, bruised lips and, on more than one occasion, tubed the goose. "Tube the goose," is ED slang for intubating the wrong pipe, the esophagus rather than the trachea.[2] Tubing the goose is easy enough to do, even if you aim at the right spot. The anatomy of the vocal cords (especially if the patient isn't properly paralyzed) can push the endotracheal tube down and into the esophagus. With time and experience I could almost immediately sense when I'd tubed the goose based on

---

2.   I am not sure how this phrase originated, but would posit that it relates to the observation that the esophagus resembles a goose's neck—long, flexible and sometimes lumpy.

the amount of resistance I felt as I advanced the tube. But those first few times, I wasn't at all sure. "Did you see the tube pass through the cords?" the attending would ask. I always thought that this was a ridiculous question, by the time I'd advanced the tube to the cords my view was pretty much obscured and the attending had to know that. But, they would ask anyway and I'd say "I think I'm in," even if I didn't, and immediately check for proper tube placement. If there was any doubt, I'd watch the patient's abdomen while a respiratory tech bagged gusts of oxygen into the tube—if the tube was in the esophagus the influx of air would cause the stomach to distend like a pregnancy. Tubing the goose was certainly embarrassing, but in most cases it wasn't detrimental to the patient if the error was rapidly identified and corrected. Unfortunately, there were exceptions to this rule and one of these was the critical trauma patient.

There were a lot of reasons why I particularly feared the trauma airway, starting with the immediacy of the situation. A patient with heart failure or pneumonia can often be observed for some time before the decision to intubate is made. This time cushion allows for mental preparation and airway assessment. Not so with some trauma patients, especially the critical ones in whom every second of resuscitation matters. Compounding the pressure of time are impediments to technique—injured patients are often bloodied and may have facial or neck trauma or missing teeth. Trauma patients transported by ambulance usually arrived in C-spine immobilization (a rigid collar that prevents flexion or extension of the neck) which is an excellent safety precaution for spinal injury but also a barrier to full airway visualization. And as the field of vision narrows, so does the margin for error.

The first "911" trauma page I received as the senior resident in charge of the airway was for a woman who had taken a shot gun blast to the head. The call came in with a five minute ETA: "65-year-old woman with severe head injury. Minimally responsive. Unable to intubate. SBP [systolic blood pressure] 160. IV established." Cursing under my breath in anxiety, I hurried to the trauma bay, donned an oppressive blue plastic gown and a welder-sized plastic faceshield and prepared my airway equipment; I checked the laryngoscope and the endotracheal tube, removed the color change detector from its packaging and drew up my medications. As I waited for the patient, my faceshield fogged with nervous breath. Just as my view of the room had misted over, the paramedics brought her in, and even through the haze, I immediately knew that I had to own this patient's airway. Her grey-tinged hair was matted with blood and her eyes held a blank stare. She was breathing on her own, but barely and with shallow chest movements. By now, the trauma bay was filled, packed with all the members of the "911" trauma activation; the ED attending, surgeons, nurses, radiology techs, the ultrasonographer and the respiratory therapist. And everyone was waiting for me, because the resuscitation started with "A" and the airway belonged to me.

Dr. Wisner, solid as a linebacker, stood in the back of the room. "Dustin," he calmly asked, "are you happy with the airway?" No I wasn't, and I said so, in a meeker fashion than I would have liked. I passed off the medications to a nurse and as she pushed them through the IV I tossed off my condensation-riddled faceshield. Sixty-some seconds later I was staring at an airway full of bubbling blood; I couldn't tell where it was coming from but it was everywhere. "What do you see?" asked the ED attending. I said nothing and re-positioned my blade. Still, I saw only frothy red. "Pulse ox is eighty-eight percent" I heard someone say and I flinched. Her blood stream was rapidly losing its oxygen. I was on the verge of panic, when my attending asked the question that surely everyone in the room was mouthing "Do you want the suction?" Yes, of course I did. He handed it to me and the bloody soup was vacuumed out with a loud whisp and there were the vocal cords in full view. I aimed right for them and although I didn't see the tube pass through, I was sure I was in. The tube misted, the lungs inflated and the color changed to yellow. "Dustin, are you satisfied with the airway?" "Airway is secure," I replied and the room reacted with a whirl of activity.

Later, I learned that the patient died—she suffered irrevocable bleeding in the brain from multiple cranial wounds. I felt ill when I heard this because the circumstances of her shooting were idiotic and would have been laughable if not so tragic. The victim had lived alone on a large parcel of land in the Sierra foothills and welcomed company whenever possible. A neighbor had occasionally been invited to hunt pheasant, quail and wild turkey on her property. Apparently as twilight fell on the fateful evening, this lonely lady ventured out to invite her neighbor to dinner. He mistook her movement for wild game and blasted away.[3]

As my first month as the owner of trauma airways progressed, it didn't take long for me to once again become numb to the tragedy and absurdity of the violence I saw. There was so much senseless tragedy; a 19-year-old girl, out with friends on her birthday, was thrown through the windshield of the car when the driver, her intoxicated boyfriend, veered into a concrete abutment. She arrived with massive swelling in the brain and little chance of survival. An inexperienced thief tried to stick up a convenience store clerk with a gun concealed in his pants

---

3.   At the time, this story seemed implausible to me. How does one mistake a grown woman for a bird? Several years later, though, after Vice President Dick Cheney made headlines by peppering a quail-shooting buddy in the face, I was forced to revise my opinion.

pocket and got an itchy trigger finger, taking out his own testicles with a bullet that then lodged in the clerk's foot. A previously healthy kid, high and psychotic on methamphetamine, saw Jesus in the headlights of the light rail train and met him, face first, decimating his jaw in the process. A neighbor enraged by a property-line dispute resorted to a baseball bat to resolve it, leaving our neurosurgeons to deal with his neighbor's cracked skull and hemorrhaging brain. A young boy playing with his father's gun mistakenly executed his younger brother with a bullet to the head.

These stories affected me in ways I probably still don't recognize, yet in that third year of residency I remained focused on airways, because my job was to be a skilled owner of airways. And over that year, I honed this skill on dozens of trauma patients, many of whom I recall only by the nature of their airway. I remember the bloody airways, the broken jaw airways, the shattered teeth airways, the dentures lodged in the pharynx airways, the difficult airways, and most vividly of all, the muffed airways. Of the latter, there were several, and each time it was something different that went wrong—challenging anatomy, a defective tube, or a goose that I just couldn't stop tubing. Fortunately, an attending was always there to assume airway ownership in my stead and none of these patients suffered from my failure. Despite this, these were the cases that haunted and distracted me. I ruminated about these airway flails for weeks and they impacted my psyche with much greater force than any of the tragic cases that traveled through the trauma bay. I suppose I should have felt guilty about this, but at the time, I didn't. It didn't even occur to me. I'd like to think that this type of tunnel focus is common among residents trying to master a critical skill. For me, at least, it took more time for the bigger picture to come into view.

◆   ◆   ◆

Nothing can justify murder, but when I later researched the Joseph Ferguson shootings, I discovered that in Ferguson's case, the circumstances of his life gave some explanation. Prior to murdering five people and severely wounding Jeffrey Mains on September 9th, 2001, Joseph lived with his father, Thomas, in a steel-bar protected brick and stucco house equipped with an armed bunker. Visitors to the Ferguson stronghold encountered an eight-foot fence adorned with barbed wire and floodlights as well as a yard full of Doberman pinschers. On the fence was a sign stating "Danger. This property protected by California Canine Security," and another featuring a picture of a Doberman and the caption "I can make it to the fence in 2.8 seconds, can you?"

Joseph Ferguson's parents divorced in 1998, a few months after his mother Susan was sentenced to a 14-year prison term at Valley State Prison for molesting Joseph and his brother. Before Joseph's mother was locked up, his father removed him from John F. Kennedy High to be home-schooled. The Ferguson men were reclusive sorts, not the types to organize a neighborhood block party or go Christmas caroling. After the shootings, one neighbor described Joseph as "one of those loner kids" and another observed that the Fergusons were "a family that wanted to be left alone." Given Joseph's upbringing and demeanor, his homicidal behavior was not a shock to some. "It doesn't surprise me," Joseph's uncle Ned Cullar said after the killings, "I fully expected to him to be one of those snipers on a rooftop someday." Next-door neighbor Will Cameron told reporters that he was "used to people getting shot" and that "in today's age, it [Ferguson's behavior] doesn't surprise me at all."

Less than a week before setting upon Sacramento with a vengeful rage, Joseph Ferguson had vented against his estranged girlfriend Nina Susu by attacking her car with an ax. Nina had subsequently told police that she thought Ferguson would kill her. Despite these and other warning signals, no one thought to separate Joseph Ferguson from the stock-pile of artillery available in and beneath his home. Perhaps Ferguson was unstoppable, so angry that he was bound to murder someone, someway, somehow. Or perhaps not.

5

A Neglected Disease

In the fall of 2004, several months after finishing my emergency medicine residency, I thought of Jeffrey Mains and wondered where he was and what he was doing. I am not sure what triggered my memory, because there were many patients that had slipped from it, but whatever it was, the recollection was clear and bittersweet. I remembered how painful his recovery had been and how it was uncertain, even when he was discharged, whether he would ever be completely well again. "You should try to find him," suggested my wife. His phone number wasn't listed in the Sacramento area, but I found some internet news reports of the shootings that mentioned Linda Mains. AT&T gave me her phone number, but when I called I only heard empty rings. Months went by and every once in awhile I thought of Mains, and at some point I began to contemplate the contradiction that his case represented. A rapid, coordinated trauma response had saved Jeffrey Mains' life but yet at the same time, his society's permissive attitude towards firearms had placed him in danger in the first place. And, of course, Mains was not alone. Despite amazing advances in the care of traumatic injury, trauma remains the leading cause of death for Americans between the ages of 1 and 44 and one-third to one-half of all trauma deaths still occur in the field—most victims succumb to injuries that not even the best trauma system on the planet could effectively treat. Did this mean, I wondered, that these deaths were inevitable and that we were bound by the maxim "shit happens" to accept a certain level of civilian casualties?

And so, as I searched for Jeffrey Mains, I concurrently researched the topic of trauma prevention and in particular the question of how best to keep innocent bystanders out of the resuscitation room. I called William Blaisdell and met him in his office at UC Davis Medical Center, where he still spent a couple afternoons a week helping David Wisner navigate administrative politics. I cracked a smile when I saw the only painting on his office wall—that of a tiger stalking in the jungle. The painting was a gift, he told me, from a former surgical resident. In an assured baritone, Blaisdell expressed pride at the progress made in the treatment of traumatic injury. "Nowadays," he told me, "we can salvage just about any patient that comes into the emergency department alive." But as incredible as this is, he explained, there is a dangerous caveat; modern trauma care has become so good that its success distracts from prevention efforts and takes away from the urgency of state-sponsored safety mandates. "I've testified and testified about auto safety and gun control," the old surgeon said wistfully, "but it is like running into a brick wall." I phoned David Wisner and he echoed his mentor's sentiments. "Prevention is an open field," he told me, "and I'm thinking passive ... cars can be made safer and guns made safer. That is where we can make the greatest progress." And while Wisner agreed that trauma surgeons had to some extent become victims of their own success, he noted that there are perceptions that form a barrier to preventive measures. One of these is that many people think of trauma as the fate of losers—of criminals, drunks and the mentally ill—and therefore not worthy of great concern. Still others feel that their freedom is threatened by mandated safety. "If you look at it from a libertarian point of view," Wisner said, "some say that there's nothing wrong with millions of people dying young from trauma, because at least they have the freedom of will to kill themselves with reckless behavior."

The more I read about the history of trauma care, the more I discovered that not only public perception, but also semantics, had heavily impacted the approach to prevention and treatment. For much of the past century in America, traumatic injuries were considered random and unpredictable "accidents," and not a disease process, like atherosclerosis or cancer, that could be studied and treated. Under this paradigm, the root causes of accidents pretty much broke down into three categories: 1) bad luck, 2) the well deserved result of stupidity, or 3) something arranged by the mafia. Prevention efforts, to the extent they existed, were predicated on warnings such as "Watch out for drunken drivers," "Don't drive too fast," or "Don't talk to strangers with loaded pistols unless they have a police badge." Fortunately for the duly warned, but not particularly safe, U.S. civilians of the 1960's, contemporaries of William Blaisdell endeavored to transform this concept of "accidents" and in particular motor vehicle "accidents." Foremost among these, was a man whose name was familiar to me: consumer activist and former presidential candidate Ralph Nader—whose 1965 book, *Unsafe at any Speed*, first brought him into the public spotlight. In this highly publicized work, Nader exposed the Big Three automaker's unconscionable resistance to instituting basic safety measures such as seat belts.[1] While Nader grabbed the headlines, a physician named William Haddon Jr. focused on overhauling the basic conceptual framework of the topic.

Before researching this book, I'd never heard of William Haddon Jr., but as soon as I pulled some articles, I realized that this was not because of his deficiencies, but rather my own. Haddon was the seminal director of the National Highway Traffic Administration and the first person to champion the concept that there's nothing "accidental" about energy transfer causing traumatic injury. It didn't matter if the energy transfer was from a high speed projectile or from rapid deceleration in a car crash, its interaction with human anatomy could be studied, and it could be modified. Accidents, Haddon argued, and car accidents especially, weren't unpredictable or random after all and so when a vehicle hit a wall it shouldn't be termed an accident but rather a *crash*. Furthermore, the outcome of that crash, in terms of human injury, was not inevitable but dependent on key variables such as speed, object malleability and passenger restraint. Haddon attempted to classify and study these variables using a conceptual tool that came to be known as Haddon's Matrix—a simple 3x3 grid identifying the factors leading to mortality and morbidity in trauma. One axis of Haddon's matrix listed three time periods: "pre-event," "event," and "post-event" and on the other were three physical components: "human," "vector" and "environment." From his matrix, Haddon extracted ten conceptual strategies for injury prevention. It would be tedious to list them all here, but it is worth noting that half of them involved the "event" phase of injury and predominantly supported the idea of "passive" injury protection—protection built into existing systems and not dependant on individual compliance. To illustrate, consider strategy number four which recommends "modifying the rate of spatial distribution of the release of the hazard from its source." This is a long-winded way of saying that an absorbed blow is less destructive, which of course is the concept supporting the use of airbags in a motor vehicle. Strategy number five suggests that we "separate in time or space the hazard being released from the people to be protected," which quite simply means that the farther you are from the action the safer you

---

1.   As you might expect, Detroit was none too pleased with Nader. In fact, General Motors (GM) hired a private investigator to tail him and dig up dirt. They found dirt; but it was smeared over their own faces. In 1966, GM president James Roche was forced to publicly apologize to Nader in front of a Congressional Committee. Nader later won a punitive lawsuit that helped jumpstart the funding he needed for years of consumer activism.

are (e.g. a pedestrian on a sidewalk is less likely to be struck by a car than one on the shoulder).

Today, Haddon's strategies sound like common sense, but what you must remember is that before him, American culture wasn't hip to prevention. Haddon's goal was to inspire a paradigm shift, to make prevention groovy—groovy in a long-winded academic way. And, I realized, in many ways he had succeeded; for today we accept that there are strategies, such as seat belts, air bags and highway speed limits that prevent or limit injury in car crashes. We recognize that crashworthy vehicles save lives and that federally-mandated improvements in car safety were the single biggest reason that U.S. car occupant fatalities (per mile of travel) decreased by two-thirds between 1964 and 1990. So while further innovation and progress is possible, there is no doubt that road safety has dramatically improved in the last 40 years. But what about other forms of traumatic injury such as gun violence? Far from getting better, I found, this is a problem that has only gotten worse.

Every year nearly 30,000 U.S. civilians are eliminated by guns, making death by firearm the fourth leading cause of preventable death for those under 65—behind heart disease, cancer and all other types of trauma combined. Homicide is a major component of the carnage—in 2001 alone there were 11,348 firearm homicides in U.S., and according to the Centers for Disease Control and Prevention (CDC), there are as many as 90,000 non-fatal gunshot wounds annually. While the total number of motor-vehicle deaths decreased 21% between 1968 and 1991 (54,862 to 43,536), firearm deaths rose 60% (23,875 to 38,317) over the same time period. Why, I wondered, has the problem of gun violence gotten worse? This is a complicated question that defies simple explanation, but it is nonetheless illuminating to view it through the lens of William Haddon Jr. Unlike many other types of trauma, injury from firearms is most effectively modified in the pre-event phase. Over fifty percent of gunshot wound fatalities are pronounced dead at the scene. This means that even if all citizens carried cell phones and could immediately call for help and even if that emergency response was proficient and a trauma center with the best possible care was nearby, post-event interventions could only decrease a community's firearm fatality rate by about half. Furthermore, event-specific interventions are limited and unlikely to garner public support. Bullets could be made with less mass and could thus be less destructive, or the momentum-producing powder charge of firearms could be reduced. But since the whole point of a gun is to be destructive, these aren't practical options. Body armor is effective (commercially available vests can stop anything up to a .38 caliber cold) and widely used by military and police personnel, but only the most paranoid civilian is likely to accept body armor as a daily wardrobe addition.

So this takes us back to the pre-event phase and the simple observation that no one dies from a shooting that doesn't happen. But is it possible to stop gun violence before it happens? Many gun control advocates say "yes" and would argue that the Jeffrey Mains shooting would never have happened if the United States, like many other civilized countries, prohibited gun ownership. There is ample evidence to support this claim; many other industrialized countries have, per capita, far less morbidity and mortality from guns than we do. There are numerous possible reasons for this discrepancy, and the shoot 'em up nature of American culture is certainly one of them, but common sense argues that lax U.S. firearm laws also play a role. A complete ban on firearms in this country, while likely to improve the problem of gun violence, is politically impossible and that's not likely to change in the near future. Are there other options? I asked William Blaisdell this question and he suggested that I speak with one of my former emergency physician colleagues at UC Davis.

"The flow of guns from manufacture to criminal use is not random," Dr. Garen Wintemute told me. "The bullet can be viewed as a pathogen, and there are patterns, analogous to a life cycle, that may allow for focused and more effective intervention." Wintemute, with his sun-browned face and sleek pony-tail, had always struck me as more of a river rafting guide than a doctor. I recalled him as an excellent physician—analytical and comprehensive—but also laid back, so much so that he was often mistaken for a lab or x-ray tech. During my residency, he had been on leave on two separate occasions to recover from an illness and although I respected his clinical skills and knew that he had done some public health research, I didn't know the extent to which he was a leader in the field of violence prevention. I was surprised to discover that he was the author of *Ring of Fire*, a book detailing how a single Southern California family monopolized the cheap handgun market for decades. He'd also been honored by *Time Magazine* as a "hero in medicine," and was currently the director of the Violence Prevention Research Program at UC Davis. When we spoke on the phone, Wintemute's voice caught inflection when I asked him about William Haddon Jr. It turns out that his own research career had been largely based on applying Haddon's conceptual framework to the problem of firearm violence. Later, when I asked him what key interventions, short of absolute gun control, could be instituted to limit gun-related injuries, he apologized and said that he would have to give me "a Haddon Matrix sort of answer," one that focused on three basic categories of pre-event interventions. Some of his proposed interventions seemed obvious to me, but I reminded myself that, much like car safety before William Haddon Jr., obvious doesn't always mean appreciated. They break down like this …

First, said Wintemute, certain people shouldn't be allowed to have guns. Foremost on this list are teenagers, criminals and the mentally ill. Even though many states have laws restricting gun ownership in these populations, they are extremely ineffective at enforcing them. A 1999 survey reported that 54% of high school students thought it would be "easy" for them to get a gun and one of Wintemute's California-based studies found that the peak age for gun possession and arrest for firearm related crimes was 18-20 years. You might expect that it would be impossible for a convicted felon to obtain a new gun, and in some instances this is true, but what about the guns he already owns? There are virtually no programs in place to divorce newly convicted criminals from their previously purchased firearms. That's fine if we're talking about someone with a life sentence, but what about a parolee with a history of violence or a youth like Joseph Ferguson who exhibits violent and erratic behavior (such as attacking a car with an ax)? In these cases all we have to rely on is the hope of successful rehabilitation and/or parental oversight.

I don't know of anyone who would like the idea of an ax-wielding car assailant or a convicted felon with a stockpile of revolvers, but as far as I'm concerned, neither of these is as scary as a paranoid schizophrenic with an empty bottle of medication and a semi-automatic. Shockingly, there is virtually no cross-referencing of state registries of the mentally ill. A florid psychotic, recently hospitalized in California could, upon his release, simply travel over a state line and purchase a gun. According to Wintemute, it is because of information-sharing failures like this that laws mandating waiting periods for gun purchases have met with mixed results. A background check without the necessary background is really no check at all.

Not only should certain civilians be kept away from guns, certain guns should be kept from civilians. These include assault weapons like the AK-47, a weapon banned by Congress[2] in 1994, and illegal in California since 1989. How did Joseph Ferguson obtain his? None of the numerous media reports covering the story answer this with certainty and Ferguson isn't around to ask, but according to Wintemute it "wouldn't have been hard" for any Californian to get an AK-47. Loopholes in federal law allowed gun manufactures to make small modifications to their assault weapons and then sell them legally at gun shows in many states, including those neighboring California. But while assault weapons like the AK-

---

2. This ban was allowed to lapse in 2004.

47 are disproportionately used in high profile shootings like Ferguson's and the Stockton school massacre,[3] overall they represent a small percentage of crime guns. Perhaps it is more important to regulate cheap and easily accessible pistols, popularly known as "Saturday night specials" that often end up in the hands of juveniles and young adults. Wintemute's research suggests that these types of guns are three times more likely to be involved in crimes, and a group of Johns Hopkins scientists estimate that Maryland's ban on Saturday night specials has resulted in a 7-12% decrease in the state's firearm homicide rate.

A third and final category of pre-event interventions involves targeted law enforcement. Comprehensive research, by Wintemute and others, has identified certain types of gun purchasers and retailers who are linked to crime guns. Emergency physician and public health researcher Arthur Kellermann has written that "... strategic firearms enforcement can block the chain of illegal events, including illegal demand, illegal supply, illegal carrying and illegal use, that leads to firearm violence." Specifically, evidence suggests that many crime guns are initially obtained from resellers who use "straw" purchases in which surrogates (without criminal records) help them purchase multiple firearms. Close tracking and investigations of transactions involving multiple firearms would help identify straw purchasers and possibly interrupt the flow of guns to criminal use. Alternatively, multiple gun purchases could be restricted (e.g. one gun per person per month), to make straw purchases more of a hassle. It also turns out that certain retailers are disproportionately tied to crime guns. Wintemute found that 10 retailers out of 3500 in California (0.2%) accounted for 13% of criminal firearms and that nationally 1% of retailers account for 57% of such guns. These statistics indicate that enforcement should be targeted towards a handful of retailers and that this could have a distinct impact on firearm crime. Prevention could also focus on high-density and high risk environments where gun violence is more likely to occur and more likely to cause harm. Certain locales—such as airports and some inner city schools—have already modulated risk by screening for firearms. These policies acknowledge the fact that disputes will occur but are often transitory. If a gun is not available in the heat of the moment the prospect of serious injury or death is diminished. If enforcement of existing laws regarding carrying firearms were stricter in high-density areas and carried enough disincentive (such as con-

3.   On January 17, 1989, 26-year old Patrick Purdy walked onto a schoolyard in Stockton, California, and opened fire with an AK-47. The shootings, which lacked an obvious motive, left five dead and wounded 30.

fiscation of the firearm), then it is reasonable to infer that fewer disagreements would end in death or serious injury.

After speaking with Wintemute I was convinced that some of America's gun violence was preventable, and preventable without strict firearm prohibition. Perhaps, with the right pre-event intervention, I concluded, Joseph Ferguson could have been stopped. If he had, it sure would have saved Jeffrey Mains a lot of suffering.

◆　　◆　　◆

Eventually, after months of intermittent effort, I tracked down Jeffrey Mains. He was in Napa, his mother told me, living with a friend, studying art, and trying to start fresh. I called Jeffrey and he said he remembered me but didn't sound completely sure. That wasn't surprising, I hadn't seen him in three years and even back then I'd never spoken with him for longer than the two minutes I'd allotted his case each morning. Nonetheless, he agreed to meet me at a coffee shop in a nearby strip mall.

Jeffrey Mains was a lot taller than I remembered, and much more robust. His 6'5" frame had filled out and his cheeks were rounded. His overall appearance was, however, softened by loose-fitting clothes and reddish-blond curls looping around a grey skull cap. The only outward sign of his ordeal was a hand tremor, a slight quake that began during his recovery. We spoke for quite a while, over hot chocolate and a tape recorder, and he told me how leaving the hospital to be at home with his mother had been immediately therapeutic. Within hours his mood brightened and within a day he was getting up from bed and walking to the dinner table. Food still passed straight through him, but at least he had had the will to eat it. Moving around continued to hurt, but at least he had had the will to walk. After a week of being under his mother's care, he returned to the medical center to see Dr. Wisner. At first, seeing him standing in the lobby, Wisner did a doubletake—like me he had never realized how tall Mains actually was. Mains remembered that Wisner told him he was doing well, that his weight was up a couple pounds and that his abdominal incisions and scars were healing nicely, with just a minimal amount of drainage from the midline scar. By then, his anxiety was waning and he was completely off the Valium and only taking Aleve for pain. Still, there was a lot to worry about, including two million dollars in medical bills, repairs to his Toyota truck, and getting healthy enough to go back to work. And, there were times when he questioned the fairness of it all.

"How could God do this to me," he recalled asking his mother, and she'd replied "I don't know why it happened, but don't blame it on God."

Eventually, as our drinks cooled and the evening wore on, Jeffrey and I caught up to the present and he told me that most of the restrictions that once ruled his life were gone—he could eat anything and do any sort of physical activity, although he had not returned to the basketball court. Tightness in his abdominal scars occasionally nagged him but he was not embarrassed to work outside bare chested. He didn't have much disposable income, but at least the insurance companies had paid off his two million dollars in medical bills. Some months after the shooting, he recalled, "I realized how much this all messed me up ... but it also forced me to focus on what I want to do with my life." Jeffrey still dreamed of teaching art, as he did before September 2001, and now he seemed determined to make the dream a reality. He was interning with Don Hatfield, a well-known and successful impressionist painter, and taking community college classes to get his bachelor's degree. "Life goes on, life does go on," he told me and he seemed hopeful; damaged but hopeful.

A year after our meeting, when I talked to Jeffrey Mains again, he seemed even better, although his career was not progressing as quickly as he would have liked. He had moved south to a small Sonoma County town called Cotati and was still in school, taking classes on Mondays and Wednesdays. The rest of the week he worked for a local butcher (a combustible chauvinist who yelled at his female employees and paid Jeffrey close to nothing) and drove to work in the same white Toyota 4x4 that had redirected Joseph Ferguson's bullet some four years before. He said he'd been writing about his ordeal for an English class and while it had been freeing, writing had also caused him to break down several times, once calling his mother in tears.

Six months later, in August of 2006, I heard from Linda Mains. Jeffrey was beset with recurrent and disabling panic attacks and bouts of severe abdominal pain. His doctor thought he was suffering from PTSD (post-traumatic stress disorder) and he was back, after many years, on anti-anxiety medication, taking as many as thirty Xanax in a week. He had quit his job in Cotati and was living at home with his mom in Sacramento, sometimes not leaving his bedroom for days at a time. I'd visited this home, a modest one with green shutters and a well-cared-for lawn, several months earlier to meet with Linda Mains and knew that the note Jeffrey had scribbled five years earlier, "We will make it," was still framed on her bedroom wall.

Linda wasn't sure what had triggered her son's setback, maybe it was the impending five-year anniversary of the shooting. Or perhaps it was the cruel realization that his dreams were proving more ephemeral than he had hoped. Whatever it was, Jeffrey wasn't ready to talk about it, at least not with me. I scheduled a meeting with him and was afraid that I'd see a man in emotional retreat, a man still suffering from the bullet's yaw. But I needn't have worried, Jeffrey Mains didn't show, and didn't call either. I don't know why but I'd like to think that it was because, five years later, he had decided once again to move on and not soak in the sour waters of the past. Or maybe the proposed date of our meeting, September 11th, 2006, carried with it too much overwhelming sadness and pain. Either, way, despite his near-miraculous salvation and nearly full recovery, the Jeffrey Mains story remained bittersweet.

6

An Unforgettable Stranger

You had a hundred billion chances and ways to have avoided today. But you decided to spill my blood. You forced me into a corner and gave me only one option. The decision was yours. Now you have blood on your hands that will never wash off ... I didn't have to do it. I could have left. I could have fled. But now I am no longer running. If not for me, for my children and my brothers and sisters that you (expletive). I did it for them ... You just loved to crucify me. You loved inducing cancer in my head, terror in my heart and ripping my soul all this time ... When the time came, I did it. I had to.

—Excerpts from the video Seung-Hui Cho sent to
NBC News, April 16th, 2007

On April 16th, 2007 I turned on the television and what I saw brought the Jeffrey Mains saga cascading back into my consciousness. Seung-Hui Cho, an angry and reclusive senior at Virginia Tech University in Blacksburg, Virginia, had committed the deadliest act of gun violence in recorded U.S. history. For days, the story was inescapable, morbidly engrossing and full of horrific stories and images; students locked in Norris Hall classrooms being picked off one by one; people leaping from second-story windows; a professor holding the door to a room shut so that his students could escape, absorbing fatal gunshots in the process; one boy protected from the assailant's bullets by a classmate's dead body; evidence of over 200 rounds of ammunition scattered throughout Norris Hall; the still photos of the killer, a young man with drawn lips and hollow eyes. Nine minutes into the carnage, just as police broke through Cho's barricade and into the building, Cho delivered his final shot, to his own temple. In all, he killed 32, injured 25 and re-ignited the smoldering issue of gun violence in America.

As I began to process the shock of the Blacksburg, Virginia tragedy, I realized how it echoed the Joseph Ferguson shootings of nearly six years before. The profile of the killers was an obvious similarity—both Cho and Ferguson were withdrawn young men with untreated psychiatric issues. While Ferguson, who by all accounts exhibited the affect and behavior of a depressed adolescent, never received entry into the mental health system, Cho had. By the fall of 2005, Cho had alarmed teachers and fellow students with his macabre writings and anti-social behavior—referring to himself as "Question Mark" and avoiding eye contact with classmates. In December of that year, two female students filed a complaint against him for harassing them with instant messages that included cryptic lines from *Romeo and Juliet*. After police warned Cho to leave the women alone, he e-mailed a roommate, stating that he might as well kill himself. This threat landed him before a community services board that declared him "mentally ill and in need of hospitalization" and then in front of state justice Paul Barnett who agreed that Cho presented "an imminent danger to himself as a result of mental illness," but nonetheless released him into involuntary outpatient therapy. In hindsight, this approach was obviously a tragic misstep; Cho never showed for his outpatient treatment. A *Washington Post* article quoted the director of the Cook Counseling Center, which was where Cho was to have sought treatment, as explaining that "when a court gives a mandatory order that someone get outpatient treatment, that order is to the individual, not an agency." Despite a state law requiring that local community service boards monitor a patient's compliance with mandatory outpatient mental health treatment, Cho slipped through the cracks and never received a full psychiatric evaluation, let alone treatment.

A second similarity between the shootings was the ease with which these two disturbed young men obtained lethal weaponry. I found an archived *LA Times* article which speculated that Ferguson, or perhaps his father, had legally obtained Chinese-made assault rifles and converted them into automatic weapons. Garen Wintemute had told me that despite California's assault weapon ban it wouldn't have been difficult for Ferguson to legally obtain these weapons in another state. On the other hand, the legality of Cho's firearm purchases had, after the shootings, become a topic of intense debate. Cho bought his guns a month apart, one through a Web site based in Wisconsin and the other at a gun shop in Roanoke, Virginia. Both times, he filled out the appropriate paperwork and underwent state and federal background checks. Cho did not offer, and the background checks did not reveal, that he had recently been adjudicated "mentally defective," and, under federal law, should have been barred from purchasing a firearm. However, under existing Virginia law, patients undergoing outpatient psychiatric therapy were not reported to the federal government's National Instant Criminal Background Check System. Two weeks after the massacre, Governor Thomas Kaine closed this loophole and mandated that reporting to the federal database be based on threat level, rather than location of treatment. "The key criteria that should trigger a report is a finding of danger," he said at a press conference. I read this announcement with skepticism, because it smelled of cover-your-ass politics, as did the talk that Congress was considering legislation that would ban the mentally ill from buying guns.

A third resemblance between the two killers was their choice of ammunition. Cho, like Ferguson nearly six years before, used hollow point bullets. Unlike Ferguson, who fired with an assault weapon and a handgun, Cho's shots were delivered exclusively by 9mm semi-automatic pistols, a Glock 19 and Walther P22. Regardless, the common choice of ammunition was a destructive one. Because hollow point bullets expand rapidly on contact, mushrooming the cavity of injury, they can cause significantly more damage than conventional, jacketed ammunition. Despite being a class of bullet banned by international treaty (The Hague Convention of 1899), some American police departments, including the NYPD, use hollow point ammunition, primarily because it delivers more effective "disabling" of hostiles and is less likely to cause secondary damage by ricocheting through one person to another. From a police perspective, this rationale made sense, but I wondered if there was a justifiable reason for public sale of hollow point ammunition. Perhaps, I discovered, there was. Some hunters who want to kill humanely choose to use hollow point ammunition rather than leave a disabled animal in the woods. But, did sportsmen need to use hand guns with hollow point bullets? What self-respecting hunter tried to off a buck with a 9mm? Why not then, ban hollow point bullets for hand guns? Sure, a motivated killer could make their own, by digging out the copper of the bullet tip, but a convenience barrier to lethality made sense. As I had already learned, however, making sense was not something that U.S. gun policy was particularly adept at.

After consulting the internet, I discovered that others had picked up on the symmetry between Ferguson and Cho. An April 2007 clip from CBS 13 in Sacramento focused, predictably, on each killer's use of video footage to chronicle his hate and to forecast its culmination. The piece replayed snippets of Ferguson's grainy six-minute video, including his boast about putting on "a hell of a show" and, his promise to, at the end of it all, "just pop" himself by sending a "bullet to the brain." Although I'd read the video transcripts many times, this was the first time I'd seen the footage. Except for one moment, when he pauses to wipe his face with his right wrist, Ferguson appears more mechanical than human: a flat-affected and murderous drone. This observation didn't surprise me, but some of the disturbing footage which followed certainly did. Against a night-time panorama of streets, cars and lights, gunshots in bursts of four and five are heard, and then the clip cuts to a man being carried by three law officers. The victim, wearing a white shirt and jeans is hauled away from a white pick-up truck with an open door and still luminescent tail lights. He is a big man, and the three officers clearly struggle to move him—holding his arms and legs as his pelvis bows in a v-configuration, nearly touching the ground. Then, without identifying the victim, the clip abruptly returns to the compassionless visage of Joseph Ferguson. Watching this, I felt a deep and cramping paroxysm seize my chest and I exhaled deeply. I hoped that Jeffrey Mains had never seen this video.

Emotionally sucker-punched by the events at Blacksburg and feeling sick because, just like the Jeffrey Mains shooting, they were preventable, I experienced an uncomfortable awakening from complacency. I was nearly three years out of residency and working in a community hospital in affluent Marin County, California. After a year or so of adjusting to a new work environment and the scary yet liberating reality of making my own clinical decisions, I had settled into a comfortable routine. Emergency medicine was, more and more, becoming just a job. I moved the patients in and out using a set of routines that I had developed for most complaints and conditions. When a nurse handed me a chart for a middle-aged patient with chest pain, I didn't need to think twice before accessing my internal protocol and scribbling out orders. Same for a young man with flank pain and blood in his urine, or a woman of child-bearing age with vaginal bleeding, or an elderly man on blood thinners who had fallen and hit his head. While moments of adrenaline still occurred, they were rare, and even the care of critically ill patients was often rote. After most shifts, I returned home tired, but far from spent; fully capable of asking about my wife's day and making simple decisions such as what to have for dinner and which DVR selection to watch afterwards. My job was still challenging, I often worked long hours and nights and was constantly multi-tasking, but it no longer sapped my life force on a daily basis. I still felt empathy for my patients, (some more than others) but slowly, shift by shift, year by year, I was building emotional defenses to protect myself from feeling too much of their pain. If I didn't do this, I rationalized, I could never survive this career for the long haul.

At my new ED, we saw trauma victims, but their injuries were of a different quality and severity than what I'd treated at UC Davis. In three years in Marin, I hadn't seen a single patient with a gunshot wound. I hadn't seen victims of baseball bats or light rail collisions or middle of the night nail-gun mishaps either. What I saw were a whole lot of recreational injuries: ankle sprains, head bonks, skinned up knees, sore wrists and bruised egos. These included mountain bikers who ate trail dirt, skate boarders who biffed and tumbled, and surfboarders whose boards jumped and popped them in the face. I sewed lacerations, reduced fractures and dislocations and prescribed copious amounts of pain medication. Occasionally, a high-speed car crash victim would be brought in and we activated our trauma protocol, but rarely were these patients seriously injured. In fact, since starting in this ED, I'd only seen one life threatening traumatic injury and this was the only time I'd felt alone without the coordinated mayhem of a Level I trauma response. A young man from the Canal district in San Rafael, one of the few rough neighborhoods in a county where the median house price tops the one million dollar mark and gun violence is as rare as a reasonably priced spa treatment, had been attacked with a machete in the middle of the night and suffered a deep arm laceration. He arrived in our ED with two paramedics desperately holding pressure on his right elbow. During transport, his wound had burst loose with arterial bleeding. I walked into Room 2 and saw a young Hispanic male who was pale, shivering and covered with sweat droplets. A river of blood ran down his arm and splattered onto the white linoleum floor. For several long seconds, the nurses looked at me with uncertainty. A trauma code had been called, but this was not the well-rehearsed environment of a Level I trauma center and our surgeon would be coming in from home rather than from around the corner. One by one, people began to move; a nurse took the blood pressure and it was 80 systolic (low); another nurse helped the paramedics with the dressing on the injured arm. IV fluid was started, oxygen applied and labs drawn. I assessed "A" and "B" of the trauma protocol and then attended to the injury. He had a full length wound just above the elbow, down to the bone. It must have been a long and sharp blade, because this man's arm was nearly severed and he was bleeding profusely, so much so that I couldn't visualize the vessels. His blood pressure remained low and he shivered like an off-kilter washer. We ordered blood and I put a blood pressure cuff above his injury and inflated it to 200. As the pressure of the cuff exceeded the arterial pressure, the bleeding slowed to a crimson ooze. Minutes later, with the patient still in obvious shock, the surgeon arrived and immediately paged for back-up.

After what seemed like an eternity, but was actually less than an hour, and multiple units of blood transfusion later, the patient left the ED for the operating room. Room 2 was left with the debris of a frenzied trauma resuscitation: discarded oxygen tubing, piles of blood soaked gauze, a Level One blood transfusion pole, rolls of the paramedic's tape, and large puddles of fresh blood. In the middle of it all was a nurse's glittery pink clog, kicked off and abandoned in the rush to move the gurney to the operating room.

The patient survived, and despite the complete disruption of his nerves, he regained some motor function in his hand. For several weeks, I felt the residual surge of fear and excitement this case stirred in me and not long afterwards I decided to return to work at UC Davis Medical Center ED as an adjunct attending. It was only one shift a month, but those days were brutally long. I would get up at 5a.m. to drive 90 minutes to Sacramento and work an often grueling 12 hour shift. Every time I got in the car to make the drive, I asked myself what I was doing and at the end of shift, after dealing with a steady stream of gore and severe illness, I'd repeat this question. But a day or so later, rested and flush with perspective, I would feel grateful to have the opportunity to work on the frontlines of medical care and to refresh my empathy reserves. It was in this spirit that I resolved to once again call on Jeffrey Mains.

In June of 2007 I emailed Jeffrey Mains, not particularly hopeful that I would receive a reply. We had been in brief email contact, but my last message, months earlier, had gone unanswered. About a month after the five-year anniversary of the shooting, I had met him and Linda Mains for dinner and confirmed the news of his downturn. We met at an Italian café in the late afternoon, a time of day at which we were the only patrons of the restaurant and were offered both lunch and dinner menus. Both Linda and Jeffrey seemed nervous, Jeffrey more so. They sat across from me at a rectangular table and Jeffrey was fidgety and restless. At one point he got up abruptly from the table to run to the bathroom and at another I noticed a fine film of sweat on his forehead. Neither mother nor son ate much. Jeffrey sipped at potato leek soup and Linda picked at a Caesar salad, and while they both answered my questions, neither expanded on their answers. Like the last time we'd met, Jeffrey's appearance surprised me—his head was closely shaven and he had a faint goatee, an inverted-T of blond on his chin. He wore thick Elvis Costello-ish brown glasses that provided an attractive contrast with his clean and recessed scalp. I noticed, for the first time, a small gap between his two upper front teeth that gave a touch of boyishness to his otherwise intelligentsia appearance. Externally, he looked good, but the internal torture was clearly still present. We spoke about his medical bills—Linda was picking up the tab for his anti-depressant and anti-anxiety medications—and he hadn't been able to afford basic follow up blood tests for his liver and gallbladder. We also spoke about the anxiety and how it could be disabling, freezing his body with tingling and an uncomfortable warmth. Jeffrey told me that it was severe enough to take him to the ED one day recently, but he calmed down when a nurse sat him in a quiet triage room and he left without a work-up. Eventually, our discussion turned from medicine and I learned about Jeffrey's departure from his apartment in Cotati, which was prompted by boredom and loneliness, and his new part-time job at the front desk of Sacramento's premier art museum, the Crocker. He was excited about the location of his job, because to work in the art world was his dream, but discouraged by the pay rate, hours and lack of health insurance. He was considering applying for state disability, based on his post-traumatic stress symptoms, but if he did this, we would have to stop working at the Crocker. He was still conflicted and still scared. After an hour or so, I noticed that Jeffrey was fidgety and when the waitress offered dessert, he quickly demurred. Already disheartened, and not wanting to push matters, I wrapped things up and we went our separate ways.

Nine months later, I was surprised when Jeffrey rapidly responded to my email: "Hey Dustin how are you doing? Well I hope," he wrote. "Things are going well around here," he continued, "it would be nice to see you if or when you come to town...." I was optimistic that Jeffrey might actually be on the rebound. It would be a couple weeks before I'd return to Sacramento and I knew there was no guarantee that, when a meeting was imminent, Jeffrey would want to re-hash old memories. In the meantime, I decided to talk to Garen Wintemute again to see if he could help me make sense of the Virginia Tech tragedy, and to inquire as to whether there was now some hope for practical gun violence prevention measures.

Dr. Garen Wintemute had just published important public health research in the journal *Injury Prevention* based on his observations of U.S. gun shows. Gun shows had long been recognized as an important source of crime guns but had never been investigated in a formal or scientific way. Increasingly, these shows were also being implicated as a major source of firearms for Mexican drug lords (an estimated 80% of illegal guns in Mexico come from the U.S.) and Canadian criminals. Motivated by the realization that "it was obvious that illegal commerce was going on at these gun shows above board and that somebody needed to tell the story," Wintemute immersed himself in the culture. Starting in April of 2005, and spanning 11 months, he attended 28 gun shows in five states: California, Nevada, Texas, Arizona and Florida. The comparison of California and the four other states allowed for a "natural experiment" between a state that regulated gun show activity (California) and four that not only did not regulate them, but were major sources of California crime guns. To carry out the experiment, Wintemute infiltrated the gun shows, subtly documenting firearm sales using a hidden camera and his cell phone (he called his voice mail to dictate observations). He paid particular attention to assault weapon sales and straw purchases (illegal surrogate purchases). What he found, in short, was that California's regulatory policies (requiring promoter and seller licensing and outlawing direct sales between private parties) worked. Despite finding that gun shows in California did not have a lower number of attendees per gun vendor compared to the other four states, Wintemute observed that California had a much lower rate of assault weapon and straw purchase sales. While he observed only one straw purchase at a California gun show, Wintemute saw 24 at shows in the other states. The manuscript describes one of these, occurring at the Florida Fairgrounds in Tampa, Florida, in March of 2006: "A woman in her 20s is purchasing an SKS rifle with a bayonet and 30-round magazine from a licensed retailer. Her male partner selects the gun, then stands 15 feet away while she completes the paperwork, undergoes a background check, and pays for the gun in cash. While waiting for the background check, he talks with the retailer about the gun, the type of case he would need and proper ammunition. He takes possession of the gun when the transaction is completed and proceeds to buy the case and ammunition." Straw purchases like these, Wintemute said, were commonly out in the open, with no evidence of attempts at concealment. "I was surprised over and over again about how out in the open all of the illegal activity was," he told me and he inferred from this observation that there was no significant effort to enforce the federal law (the Gun Control Act of 1968) banning straw purchases of firearms.

I asked Wintemute about the reaction to his study and received a measured response. Some in law enforcement, especially at the Bureau of Alcohol, Tobacco and Firearms (ATF) were very excited, but others quickly became defensive. He described blogs on which gun enthusiasts denigrated his results and referred to him as a "boob," a "leftard," and a "douchebag." On the Web and at some gun shows, "wanted" posters had appeared with Wintemute's photo and the warning that the man pictured was an anti-gun "researcher" known to stalk gun shows. His methods and credibility came under attack and the National Rifle Association (NRA) and others dismissed the existence of a gun show problem all together. I found one blogger from Kennesaw, Georgia, "The Conservative Scalawag," whose posts captured the mentality of some in the pro-gun camp. "Once again here is some boob, propagating the gun show loop[hole] myth," he wrote. "I'm not saying there aren't irresponsible people or unscrupulous people at gun shows. But, I doubt however if they're selling full auto AK-47s … To me gun show are a piece of Americana and it is what makes the nation so great. To loss them is to loss our identity as a free people."[1] Elsewhere, at the debate between Democratic presidential candidates sponsored by YouTube, a man from Michi-

---

1. Grammatical errors belong to the Scalawag

gan, while cradling his assault rifle, expressed concern that Democrats would take away his "baby." "If that's his baby," retorted Senator Joeseph Biden, "he needs help." The mentality of pro-gunners like this was perfectly captured by Erik Larson in his 1994 book *Lethal Passage; How the travels of a single handgun expose the roots of America's gun crisis*: "Theirs is a reflexive opposition based on the rather paranoid belief that any step towards firearms regulation must necessarily take us one more step down the road to federal confiscation of America's guns and, willy-nilly from there, to tyranny and oppression."

I had read Wintemute's paper before talking with him and knew that it had garnered coverage in the *USA Today* and *The Christian Science Monitor*. I was hopeful that it, along with the memory of the Blacksburg killings, had sparked interest among saner minds in Washington, D.C. The message, after all, that regulation without prohibition can diminish illegal gun commerce, ought to be of some importance. Wintemute was pessimistic. An unnamed Senator was interested in introducing a bill to regulate gun shows and close the "gun show loophole" that allowed unlicensed gun dealers to make illegal private party sales, but the prospects of getting anything passed were poor. Congress' focus, he informed me, was to address public concern about the Virginia Tech shootings by passing an NRA-supported bill regulating the sale of guns to the mentally ill. This, we both agreed, was a necessary reform, but one that attempted to plug a boulder-sized problem with a pebble. For certain, legislation that provided incentives for states to share criminal and mental health records with the feds would be useful—at the time of the Virginia Tech Shootings, only 22 states (including Virginia) supplied such information to the federal government. But why, I asked, limit reform to the mentally ill, a diverse population who account for only a small percentage of violent crimes? But, I needn't have asked, I knew that the answer was because the issue of gun control was too emotionally charged and that the nation did not have the stomach to seriously address the issue of gun violence. This of course has been the case for quite a long time. A certain subset of the American public is so invested in the issue that public policy has evolved to the point that not only is banning guns off the table, but studying the problem of gun violence is almost impossible. Wintemute told me that he was one of less than a dozen public health researchers in the country studying the problem of gun violence. As of 1996, the CDC was forbidden from funding any studies that could be construed to support gun control and between 1973 and 2002 the National Institutes of Health (NIH) had only funded two grants addressing injury prevention from firearms. In the last several years, Congress has passed the NRA-backed Tiahrt amendment, ostensibly to protect law enforcement (but actually to protect gun manufacturers), that makes it a crime for law enforcement to share information on sources of crime guns unless they are directly involved in an investigation involving a specific gun. This in a country that is home to 220 million guns and, each year, witnesses 4 million gunshots and 430,000 gun-related crimes (including 11,000 homicides). Reflecting on this, I was reminded of a quote from the National Academy of Sciences' landmark publication *Accidental Death and Disability: the Neglected Disease of Modern Society*: "The long-term solution to the injury problem is prevention and the major responsibility for accident prevention rests not with the medical profession, but with educators, industrialists, engineers, public health officials, regulatory officials and private citizens." This was written in 1966 and preceded a remarkable transformation in the safety of our nation's roads that was defined by public consensus on what constituted the best interests of the country; a transformation driven by an approach to accidents that treated them as a disease, a disease that could controlled. Nearly 40 years later, the quote from the National Academy of Sciences is still applicable—only now to the problem of gun violence. Maybe, I thought, Wintemute's study would be the first step towards sensible gun policy, but perhaps it would just add fuel to the flames of conflict and debate.

◆   ◆   ◆

It was a sweltering July day when I drove up to Sacramento to meet with Jeffrey Mains. Driving in our 1993 Plymouth minivan, which no longer had functional AC, I tried to imagine what Jeffrey would look and sound like. It was difficult, though, because the heat distracted me and I repeatedly reached my hand into the cooler on the passenger's seat in order to feel something refreshing against my skin. By the time I neared Sacramento, I was damp from sweat and feeling detached. In the eastern foreground, a large bank of clouds rose from the valley, mountains of white. Straight ahead, I imagined the two claws and mouth of a crab emerging from the cloud line, trying to push free. I considered, for a moment, if that crab would work as a metaphor for Mains, and then decided that a story like his was too complex for that.

We met up that evening. It was still hot, but had cooled some, enough to clear my head. I saw Jeffrey walking down the sidewalk along Folsom Boulevard—a tall and confident walk. Physically, he looked similar to when I had seen him last, he was wearing green cargo shorts, a white shirt and flip flops and sporting close cut blond hair, dark-rimmed glasses and a hint of a goatee. His affect, however was fresh and assured. We walked together down Folsom Boulevard to East Sacramento Hardware so that Jeffrey could pick up some electrical tape. He was working full time, he told me, at the Crocker Art Museum but the pay wasn't great, so he did some work for a contractor friend on the side. The day before he had mistakenly sawed through the cord of his power saw on the job. He didn't seem too perturbed about the mishap and was shrugging it off with a 'no worries' attitude. We traded home improvement disaster stories as we waited in line at the hardware store before we were interrupted by a middle-aged woman who asked Jeffrey if he knew where the sprinkler heads were displayed. He considered the question for several seconds before admitting that he didn't know. When the customer persisted with her query, he politely explained that he actually didn't work at the store and was just waiting for the cashier. Then he gave me a grin.

I had planned for us to eat at the same Italian café, but it had closed early that afternoon because their dishwasher was MIA, so instead we sat outside a small taco stand several blocks down from the hardware store. We were the only customers and had the outdoor tables and mist fan all to ourselves. I had brought a notebook with a list of questions—both medical and personal—but I felt uncomfortable disrupting the easy flow of our stroll from the hardware store. I resolved to lock the details of the conversation into my memory and at first was successful; Jeffrey was still living at home with Linda, but now was doing so in part to help her out by paying rent. The job at the Crocker was going well and there was a good chance he'd get a city position as the director of art placement with them. If that happened, he'd have health insurance, but even if not he was now five years past his injury and eligible for an affordable rate. His anxiety was much better and he rarely required Xanax. His re-routed guts were working well and while he still hadn't received any follow-up testing, he wasn't experiencing any intestinal discomfort. Jeffrey told me that he was starting to paint again, mainly still lifes and in black and white, and his work at the Crocker had helped him believe that he had the ability to produce art work that people would buy. He had some ideas for figures, he told me, simple scenes like a couple sitting at the bar or a couple of dudes at a taco joint. Jeffrey had been dating a career-oriented woman for several months and now spent most nights at her place. He seemed happy with the relationship and I could tell that it gave him footing. After awhile, I began to lose some details of the conversation, as we moved beyond bullet points to a back-and-forth about art, writing, books, and careers. I found myself describing my own evolution into a part-time writer and lamenting the difficulty of finding the time and inspiration to pursue this interest. We talked about how John Grisham, when he worked as a lawyer before becoming a best-selling author, used to wake up at 5a.m. to dedicate one hour to writing and that over several years he had written his first novel this way. We also traded ideas on how Jeffrey could cash in on his artistic talents with a commercially hot image, perhaps, I suggested, one that captured the surreal nature of the annual Burning Man festival in the Nevada desert. After we'd finished our burritos and started to notice the expectant looks from the taco shop attendant waiting to close down, I realized that this wasn't an interview anymore, it was two 30ish-year-old guys with similar interests hanging out and shooting the shit. This story had progressed far beyond a young doctor and the patient that he saw for two minutes each morning, it was now about the life that lay beyond the bullet's yaw.

Select Bibliography

American College of Surgeons Committee on Trauma. *ATLS; Advanced trauma life support program for doctors: student course manual.* 7th Edition. Chicago: American College of Surgeons, 2004.

Blaisdell FW, Grossman M. *Catastrophes, epidemics and neglected diseases. San Francisco General Hospital and the evolution of public care.* San Francisco: The San Francisco General Hospital Foundation, 1999.

Bureau of Alcohol Tobacco and Firearms. *Commerce in Firearms in the United States.* Washington, DC: Bureau of Alcohol, Tobacco and Firearms; 2000.

Diehl D. The emergency medical services program. In: Isaacs SL, Knickman JR, ed. *To improve health and health care 2000: the Robert Wood Johnson Foundation anthology.* San Francisco: Josey Bass Publishers, 2000.

Duval MK. *Health care's hidden crisis.* Journal of the American College of Emergency Physicians. Jan/Feb:14-16 (1972).

Franklin J, Doelp A. *Shock-trauma.* New York: St Martin's Press, 1980

Kellermann AL. *Treating gun violence before the 911 call.* Annals of Emergency Medicine. 43:743-745 (2004).

Larson E. *Lethal passage: how the travels of a single handgun expose the roots of America's gun crisis.* New York: Crown Publishers, 1994.

Mattox KL, Feliciano DV, Moore EE, ed. *Trauma.* 4th Edition. New York: Mcgraw-Hill, 2000.

National Center for Health Statistics. Available at: http://www.cdc.gov/nchs/fastats/injury.htm.

National Academy of Sciences National Research Council. *Accidental death and disability: the neglected disease of modern society.* Washington, DC: National Academy of Sciences, 1966.

O'Neill B. *Accidents or crashes: highway safety and William Haddon, Jr.* Contingencies. Jan/Feb:30-32 (2002).

Robertson LS. *Groundless attack on an uncommon man; William Haddon, Jr, MD.* Injury Prevention. 7:260-262 (2001).

Webster DW, Vernick JS, Hepburn LM. *Effects of Maryland's law banning "Saturday night special" handguns on homicides.* American Journal of Epidemiology. 155:406-412 (2002).

Wintemute GJ. *Ring of fire: the handgun makers of Southern California: a report from the Violence Prevention Research Program.* Sacramento: The Program, 1994.

Wintemute GJ. Gun shows across a multistate American gun market: observational evidence of the effects of regulatory policies. Injury Prevention. 13:150-156 (2007).

Wintemute GJ, Parham CA, Beaumont JJ, Wright M, Drake C. *Mortality among recent purchasers of handguns.* New England Journal of Medicine. 341:1583-1589 (1999).

Wintemute GJ, Romero MP, Wright MA, Grassel KM. *The life cycle of crime guns: a description based on guns recovered from young people in California.* Annals of Emergency Medicine. 45:733-742 (2004).

Zink BJ. *Anyone, anything, anytime; a history of emergency medicine.* Philadelphia: Mosby, 2006.

About the Author

Dustin W. Ballard received his MD from the University of Pennsylvania and completed his residency training in emergency medicine at the UC Davis Medical Center in Sacramento, California. Dr. Ballard's writing credits include co-authorship of the award-winning travel narrative *A Blistered Kind of Love: One Couple's Trial by Trail* (Mountaineers Books, 2003) and contributions to *Hoops Nation* (Owl Books, 1998). He currently works as an emergency physician in Northern California where he lives with his wife Angela, daughter Hayley, and Labrador retriever Gary.

978-0-595-47648-0
0-595-47648-1

www.ingramcontent.com/pod-product-compliance
Lightning Source LLC
Chambersburg PA
CBHW051212050326
40689CB00008B/1288